Global Health Nursing

7/16

Christina A. Harlan, MA, BSN, RN, teaches in the School of Nursing at the University of North Carolina at Chapel Hill. Her teaching and clinical experience is in global public health. Ms. Harlan has worked as a public health nurse in Latin America and the Caribbean as well as in multi-ethnic, multilingual, rural and urban communities in the United States. She is a lifelong learner of languages with primary proficiency in Spanish. Ms. Harlan is the co-author of several Spanish-language and culture publications.

Global Health Nursing
Narratives From the Field

Christina A. Harlan, MA, BSN, RN

Editor

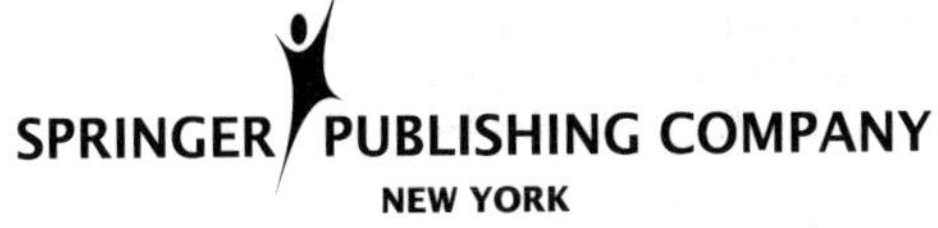

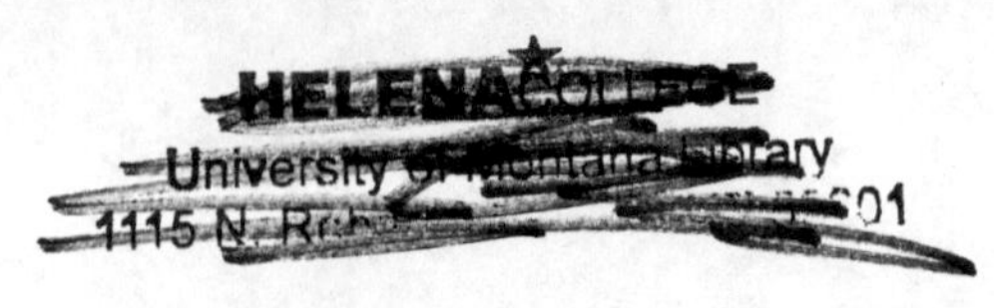

Springer Publishing Company, LLC
11 West 42nd Street
New York, NY 10036
www.springerpub.com

Acquisitions Editor: Joseph Morita
Production Editor: Brian Black
Composition: diacriTech

ISBN: 978-0-8261-2117-2
e-book ISBN: 978-0-8261-2118-9

14 15 16 17 / 5 4 3 2 1

Library of Congress Cataloging-in-Publication Data

Global health nursing (Harlan)
Global health nursing : narratives from the field / Christina A. Harlan, editor.
p. ; cm.
Includes bibliographical references and index.
ISBN 978-0-8261-2117-2 -- ISBN 978-0-8261-2118-9 (e-book)
I. Harlan, Christina A., editor. II. Title.
[DNLM: 1. Nursing Care. 2. Cross-Cultural Comparison. 3. Internationality. 4. Nurse's Role. 5. Transcultural Nursing. 6. World Health. WY 100.1]
RT34
610.73092'2—dc23
2014020374

Printed in the United States of America by Edwards Brothers Malloy.

The past couple of decades have seen the rise of a new and deepening interest in global health: efforts to bring the fruits of modern medicine to those living in settings of privation. Nurses have been the stalwarts and the backbone of global health care delivery, serving as a point of first contact for many of our patients, from Haiti to Rwanda, and offering the promise of continuing care rooted in a respect for and a commitment to health equity. Nurses' expertise and perspective are essential to the development of sound health policy and practice, but their voices too often go unheard. The narratives in this book offer rare and much-needed insight into the lived experiences and contributions of the largest cadre of global health workers: the nurses who have dedicated their careers and their lives to serving the world's poor.

Paul Farmer, MD, PhD
Kolokotrones University Professor,
Harvard University
Co-Founder, Partners in Health

Such compelling narratives in a series of clear and intimate journeys, Global Health Nursing: Narratives From the Field *is a testament to the best of nursing practice today; improving and achieving health equity by caring for our neighbors—whether next door or around the world.*

Karen Mountain, MBA, MSN, RN
Chief Executive Officer
Migrant Clinicians Network

In this engaging collection, nurses who have lived and worked in the far-flung corners of the world tell their personal stories and give the reader a vivid picture of the many opportunities that await health professionals willing to serve where the need is great, the conditions demanding, and culture unfamiliar. They reveal what led them on the path to global nursing, what challenges they met, and what they learned along the way. In these inspiring essays, written with great humility, the nurses open their hearts to the reader and share what they were able to give to their patients, what they received, and how the experience of global nursing changed and enriched their lives.

Ruth Stark, PhD, NP, RN
author of *How to Work in Someone Else's Country* (2011)

Contents

Contributors

Tina Anselmi-Moulaye, MSN, CNM
Sidra Medical and Research Center
Doha, Qatar

Carole F. Bennett, PhD, APRN, PMH-CS
Assistant Professor
School of Nursing
Georgia Southern University
Statesboro, Georgia

Naomi J. Blackman-Abdellaoui, BSN, RN
Field Nurse
Médecins Sans Frontières
New York, New York

Jacqueline Boulton, MSc, RGN, RM, PGCAP, FHEA, Diploma in Tropical Nursing
Tutor in Adult Nursing
Kings College
London, England

Jane Calthrop, MEd, BS, BSN, RN
University of North Carolina Healthcare
Chapel Hill, North Carolina

Marie Collins Donahue, MPH, MS, CPNP-PC, RN
Pediatric Nurse Practitioner
University of North Carolina Children's Hospital
Chapel Hill, North Carolina

Jennifer Foster, CNM, MPH, PhD
Associate Clinical Professor of Nursing
Associate Professor of Global Health
Associate Faculty in Anthropology
Nell Hodgson School of Nursing
Emory University
Atlanta, Georgia

Anna Freeman, MPH, BSN, RN
Field Nurse
Médecins Sans Frontières
New York, New York

Jenny Hartsell, RN
Executive Director and Founder
Shared Beat
Boerne, Texas

Teresa Johnson, BSN, RN
Heartcry Missionary Society
Radford, Virginia

Trevor C. Johnson, MA, BSN, RN
Heartcry Missionary Society
Radford, Virginia

Linda Joseph, BSPH, NCSN, RN
Orange County Schools
Hillsborough, North Carolina

Christina Martinez Kim, MSN, BSN, BS, RN
Psychiatric Mental Health Nurse Practitioner
Duke University Health System
Durham, North Carolina

Candace Kugel, MS, FNP, CNM
Clinical Specialist
Migrant Clinicians Network
Austin, Texas

Kim L. Larson, PhD, RN, MPH
Associate Professor
College of Nursing
East Carolina University
Greenville, North Carolina

Naomie Marcelin, RN
Clinical Nurse Administrator
Lead Nurse Educator
Partners In Health/Zanmi Lasante
Hôpital Universitaire de Mirebalais
Mirebalais, Haiti

Ruth-Anne McLendon, BSN, RN
Student
School of Nursing
University of North Carolina at Chapel Hill
Chapel Hill, North Carolina

Pamela A. McQuide, PhD, BA, BSN, RN
Chief of Party
IntraHealth International
Klein Windhoek, Namibia

Jana Mervine, BSN, RN
Executive Director and Founder
Among the Stars, Inc.
Miami, Florida

Laura Calamos Nasir, PhD, MSN, FNP, FHEA
Senior Lecturer
College of Nursing, Midwifery and Healthcare
University of West London
London, England

Mike Olufemi, MS, MBA, BS, BSN, RN
Duke Regional Hospital
Durham, North Carolina

Joyce Smith, HV, MPHIL, RN
Human Resources Specialist (retired)
World Health Organization
Lombok, Indonesia

Margaret Thornton, MSN, BSN, RN
Volunteer (retired)
Pine Street Inn
Boston, Massachusetts

Foreword

Our stories are our legacies. The nurses who share their stories in this book come from a variety of backgrounds, ages, specialties, motivations, and experiences. There are stories from students, new nurses, experienced nurses, nursing faculty, and nurse researchers. Some of the nurses in the book did not start out with a desire to work globally, others went into nursing to be able to do precisely that, and others intended to go for one trip and kept going back. Confronting severe poverty, violence, and gender-based inequities is difficult. Sadly, lack of clean water, plentiful food, or safe sleeping spaces is commonplace for many people in the world. Seeing and experiencing these things first hand can be life changing for an outsider. Many contributors to this book experienced frustration, cultural discordance, difficulty, and utter joy.

The confluence of opposite emotions is common in nursing, and nowhere is it more distinctive than in global nursing. Each story represents a journey for the nurse and for those with whom she or he has worked. We will benefit by hearing from nurses who took a risk and shared honestly what they saw, heard, and felt. Nurses from resource-rich settings such as the United States are represented, and, thankfully, we also hear the voices of nurses on the other side of the story, those who are the beneficiaries of our "help." This opportunity is rare and provides a richness that is not often revealed.

The relationship is complicated; we hear the frustration, sadness, and feelings of being overwhelmed from the nurses who have traveled with the best intentions to "do good." We also hear the challenges of being on the beneficiary side of that help; when it can be painful, infuriating, and insulting to have nurses come into your country with preconceived, colonialist, and even voyeuristic notions about the situation, your training/education, and your culture. It is also apparent that there are overwhelming feelings of gratitude for the compassionate and skilled nurses who have traveled to help during times of acute and chronic disasters.

The most successful scenarios in global nursing are where nurses approach their traveling work with humility, respect, and sincere appreciation for what they will be learning from their global colleagues. Skills transfer and knowledge sharing is best done after the identification of needs by those who are being helped—the nurse, the patient, and the community. Regardless of what skills are brought, most nurses are not experts in nursing in a country foreign to them. The most experienced specialty-trained critical care nurse will be completely ineffective if he or she cannot translate that knowledge into a local context. There may be limited, if any, medications, electricity, water, staff, and a limited or nonexistent health infrastructure. Colleagues in these countries are the key to bridging that gap. These nurse colleagues will also be the ones who will remain when others are long gone; an important reality that one should never forget.

I am fortunate to have nursing colleagues from all over the world at Partners In Health (PIH) who are experts from Haiti, Rwanda, Malawi, Navajo Nation, and beyond. My job is to work side by side with them—to listen, learn, share knowledge, and respond to their identified needs. The best advice I received when I began working in Africa more than 15 years ago was from an experienced global nurse who cautioned me to listen more than to talk and to be okay with the silence—advice I still try to follow every day.

Nurses represent the largest cadre among health workers. We work in every conceivable setting, from remote mountainous regions of Lesotho to the most populated cities of the world. Nurses are underrepresented in leadership, at policy tables, in health program decision making, and governmental bodies, in both resource-rich *and* resource-limited settings. There is a growing appreciation for the important role of nurses, midwives, and the slowly increasing cadre of advanced practice nurses. The challenge is to harness that appreciation and advocate for increased inclusion of nurses at every level of the health care delivery system. We are our own best promoters; it is our responsibility to illuminate the voices of our global nursing community.

Nurses know what they need to provide the best care for their patients: access to formal education, skills enhancement, and career development to address the complexities of health care delivery. Our patients need access to a well-educated multidisciplinary team of health care providers who have the necessary tools to provide care. They also need the basic tenets of human rights: water, food, security, and access to health care. We must work together to address social determinants of health such as poverty and lack of education.

These stories—in which nurses bear witness to the best and worst in the world—are important reading for all nurses, student nurses, and potential nurses. This book is about nurses, our profession, and our ability to provide compassionate care in unfamiliar, sometimes dire, and even desperate environments. What we learn is that the art and science of nursing can transcend geography, language, and cultural differences if approached with humility, shared respect, and combined effort. The voices in these stories also provide a window into global nursing for our colleagues, families, and friends who may not understand the drive, motivation, and passion that we all have to be able to work in settings not our own. It is often hard to describe what we see and what we do—it can be too close, too raw, too emotional, or too exhausting to explain. Now we can let each other's voices tell our stories.

Sheila M. Davis, DNP, ANP-BC, FAAN
Chief Nursing Officer
Partners In Health

Preface

My dream for many years was to write—or more accurately, to convince a colleague to write—a global health nursing book. There had been no progress on either front until it finally dawned on me that no task is too daunting if it is shared. I am a beader. I take unique handcrafted beads and string them into beautiful works of art. I've approached my task as editor in the same way. To paraphrase 3M's advertisements—I didn't write it . . . I made it better!

My background is in public health nursing with graduate studies in anthropology. The triangulation of nursing, public health, and anthropology has given me a rich life, personally and professionally. As I worked on edits for this book, I thought about my own experiences and recognized parallels in the road I followed with that of my colleagues.

When I was 7 years old, my grandparents boarded a tramp steamer in New York Harbor and embarked on a 2-year trip around the world. My parents mounted a large map on my bedroom wall on which I placed pins as I followed their journey through letters home. Thus began my passion for travel and languages.

I trace my interests in nursing and public health to when I was a child living in Alaska and my sister and I were diagnosed with hepatitis A. It seems that the Native Alaskans in the community were blamed for the epidemic. That was my introduction to the concept of social determinants of health, although it would be many years before I made the connection.

After nursing school, I joined the Peace Corps and was assigned to Brazil. While there, I visited a psychiatric hospital that made me feel I had walked into the Middle Ages—stone walls, patients without clothing eating on tin plates on the floor. I felt angry and helpless and at the same time realized a great appreciation for Dorothea Dix.

I worked as a home health nurse in the mountains of Puerto Rico in order to improve my Spanish. I had come from Boston, where there is a large Puerto Rican community, and planned to return. My "ticket" into my patients' world was my nursing skills, evaluating a wound, checking blood pressure, and teaching about diabetes. I worried they would feel disadvantaged by having a *gringa* nurse who bumbled her way through their language. Apparently my patients and their families understood that by helping me with my Spanish, they, in turn, would be helping other Puerto Ricans living in Boston. The sense of reciprocity was strong and I felt a mutual value in what we could each contribute to the other.

While working at a health center serving migrant farmworkers in North Carolina, I was asked to explain the behavior of a "crazy Haitian lady." My husband comes from Haiti so the staff of the center at which I worked thought I might have some insight into why a patient apparently tried to give away her newborn baby to one member of the hospital staff. When the staff person declined the offer, the woman "lost it"—hence the label "crazy." I don't know what was going on in her mind. But I do know that in many societies when parents feel they cannot care for their children, they "give" their children to persons of perceived higher status. Within the realities of their lives, these parents believe they are doing the very best they can for their children. As folks at the health center recalled the event, I couldn't help but wonder how they might have handled the situation differently if they had interpreted it as an adoption story rather than simply that of a "crazy lady."

Once, I was invited to Bolivia to provide health education to women in prison. It was disturbing to learn that many of the women were there because of nonpayment of debts. Their children lived in the prison—going out to school each day and returning "home" to their mothers each evening. Contrast that experience with my visit to a home for the children of people diagnosed with leprosy. The children had been removed from their birthplace—a leper colony on an island off the coast of Brazil—to grow up separated from their parents.

I remember going out to dinner in Haiti with a group of my husband's friends. The conversation at the table ebbed and flowed in

French, Haitian Creole, English, and Spanish because there was no one common language among the group. My French and Creole are not strong. So my husband carefully repeated to me what was being said while remaining in the language being spoken. By "dumbing down" the language, I could understand what was happening while at the same time keeping the conversation going without reverting to English. When I worked as a home health nurse in Massachusetts I alternated between Spanish and Portuguese during the day as I visited Puerto Rican and Cape Verdean patients. In North Carolina, while working with migrant farmworkers, I went back and forth between Spanish and Haitian Creole. I imagine languages sitting on railroad tracks in my brain. I visualize railroad lines switching gears from one language track to another the way a train does. Sometimes I have to pause for a moment so that the switch goes smoothly. Most times, I don't even realize it is happening.

As a nursing instructor, I have had the privilege of facilitating global experiences for students, through spring-break trips to Guatemala and through a series of global health courses that I teach. One such course offers our rising seniors an opportunity to travel over the summer to a country of their choice, for a length of time of their choice, to volunteer in a health care agency of their choice. The course is taught asynchronously, online. It represents a unique model among nursing schools. Typically, a faculty member travels with a group of students to a known location. In this case, students have a great deal of autonomy in planning their experience, which they highly value. Every nursing program includes objectives for teaching critical thinking skills and leadership. This course, Practicum in Nursing: Global Health Experience, provides a structure in which students meet these objectives organically. Students are often curious about my work history because they want to understand what it takes to develop a career in global health. My response to them is this book.

I have had the pleasure of working with many gifted colleagues over the years. At the start of this project I reached out to a number of them, asking them to contribute their stories and to assist me in identifying others who could do so as well. The result is a collection of narratives written by nurses who represent a range of expertise, working in diverse regions of the world. I recognize that there are many skilled nurses contributing to global health who are not represented here.

To get started, I asked the contributors to be reflective and practical as they described their work in global health. I asked them to say something about their background and motivation for working globally. I also asked them to consider ethical, cross-cultural, and/or sustainability issues encountered and to describe how they handled those situations. Finally, I asked them to give advice to other nurses who may be considering global health work. They took me at my word. Although each nurse followed the same guidelines, he or she approached his or her story in different ways. The end result is this compelling collection.

For the purposes of this endeavor, global health nursing is defined as work in a country different from that of the author, and/or work with vulnerable populations at home. By including material from our home countries an important point is made: "global is local." Contributors describe assumptions that were challenged and lessons learned that guide their work in settings with people whose life experience is greatly different from their own.

With this collection of narratives we have an opportunity to hear the voices of nurses for whom global health nursing is a passion. Nurses new to the profession describe their student experiences, and new graduates discuss their strategies for developing appropriate skills. More seasoned nurses reflect on the trajectory of their careers that led to significant contributions in global health practice, consultation, and research. Throughout the book, nurses describe how they encourage the next generation of nurses through their teaching and mentoring. Their stories are written with compassion, humor, and insight.

We all began our careers as students. Travel abroad for students in the health professions is not just a wonderful personal adventure but is also important to our professional development. Global health experiences will inform a students' practice for a lifetime, as demonstrated in the writings of many contributors to this work.

To further illustrate my point, the final chapter was written by a former student who, after traveling abroad for the global course described earlier, expressed an interest in taking lessons learned to a higher level. Inclusion of her chapter, along with those of several other students, is a clear indication that the future of global health nursing is bright.

I believe this book will be of interest to young people who are considering nursing as a career, to professional nurses who hope to contribute their knowledge and skills to improving the health of vulnerable populations, to nursing students who dream of working globally, and to faculty who seek creative ways to prepare their students for work in a global context.

This book will also be helpful to health professionals who work with diverse populations, including recent immigrants. Greater knowledge regarding health status and health systems in other countries enhances our ability to appropriately provide care to patients and communities globally as well as locally.

No one person could have written this book. They say it takes a village to raise a child. In this case it took a village to write a book. I thank everyone who shared their heartfelt narratives.

Christina A. Harlan

Acknowledgments

I wish to acknowledge colleagues at the University of North Carolina at Chapel Hill School of Nursing who, for many years, have partnered with me to identify creative strategies for responding to the global health interests of our students, in particular: Gwen Sherwood, Beverly Foster, Katherine Moore, and Janna Dieckmann. I also want to thank Marilyn Oermann for her guidance in navigating the world of publishing; Alisa Watson-Mebane for her copyediting skills; and my division chair, Cheryl Jones, for her enthusiastic endorsement of my interest in gathering narratives to illuminate the global health work of nurses.

Several contributors to this collection were especially supportive of my endeavor: Laura Nasir, Christina Martinez Kim, Anna Freeman, Naomi Blackman-Abdellaoui, and Kim Larson. With their encouragement and our collective networking skills, I was able to identify an impressive group of nurses for this project.

A special note of love and thanks goes to my parents Dan and Mary Ann; my husband Dimi (aka Edwin); and our children Edwige, Lucas, and Noël, with whom "global is local" has been a lived experience.

Prologue

How Vision Forms

She sits, in my mind's eye, on that stone step in front of the hut where she must have slept. Smiling wryly at my camera she wore red sweat pants and a t-shirt while the other ladies were dressed in threadbare and faded saris. She had a smart spark in her eyes and laughed easily as she chatted in broken English with us American students about marriage, sex, and Kathmandu—as if it were all so regular, as if she weren't so odd compared to the other people in this Gurung village. We were one walking-day away from any sort of town, and in this tiny Himalayan village she was a rarity—a single woman with no children. I was 21 and traveling abroad to study Hindu mythology and literature—she seemed so old and wise in the ways of the country and yet now I must guess she wasn't more than 20 herself. The villagers spoke of Nepal like a distant land and Kathmandu like an exotic country. "Capital city" and "nation" were concepts they had little use for, and this girl, Sonu, was an outsider though she was from a town only a few miles away.

Settling into the village I was directed to a little corner of my own. I slept in my sleeping bag in the barn where grain was stored. They must have told me the names of things as they directed me there, but my Nepali language hadn't gotten past learning numbers. The family hosting me slept in the single bed in the single room on the floor below mine; the parents and their three girls, the youngest knowing more English words than I knew in Nepali.

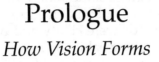

I woke the next morning to a stunning sunrise—and a row of grinning kids who had watched me sleep. They giggled when I brushed my hair, were stunned when I brushed my teeth, and when they all rushed to grab at my brushes, I decided it was time to explore. If their local visitor Sonu was different, then I was clearly an exotic novelty. The kids led me around the village consisting of maybe a couple dozen huts, showing me their school with great pride—one room with a tin roof, which was more than most villages could boast. As we walked, the children took turns running ahead, telling me about the site, and taking my hand, talking and laughing nonstop. Understanding little, I tried to take it all in and guess at the patterns and meanings.

Then she was there again, Sonu, in a little room by the big room called the school. The kids were chatty and uninterested, but I was captured. Sonu was weighing babies on a huge scale, large enough for a bursting watermelon. She unwrapped the baby and put him or her on the scale, as the nervous mother looked on. Sonu marked a number on the wall of the hut in dark kohl, smudged black just like the heavy eyeliner around the babies' eyes, put there to ward off evil spirits. Was she a nurse? Was this some kind of health promotion center in such a little faraway place?

I was there to ask about the stories of Rama, images of Ganesh, to locate, I thought, old dusty tomes, or scrolls, or tablets about the ancient gods. But it was no use. There were no such fantastical items. And few could read or write in all the country. The kids everywhere asked for pencils "*Collom cha*?" But they had no paper. I soon realized I would be just as lost asking my American neighbor about the history and cultural significance of the Christmas tree. It might be a lovely item, but not the important part of the story. In a town of huts without electricity or running water, storing esoteric ideas was unusual and unnecessary.

I felt my love of books slipping away, replaced by a new feeling—a need, actually—to be able to give some knowledge back. I watched them, they watched me. But was there something I could *do*? My eyes opened wider . . .

I traveled for many weeks in Nepal and across the Himalayas, but after meeting Sonu it seemed that every kid was asking for antibiotics or Band-Aid™. Leprosy-scarred beggars sat on every corner and a cure for diarrhea was the conversation started by every traveler. My search for fascinating cultural tales shifted to an interest in using my hands, to learning how to respond to the seemingly endless number of bicycle crashes in the crowded bazaars. And a vision grew of how a young woman with just a little bit of daring might be able to make a difference.

Laura Calamos Nasir, PhD, MSN, FNP, FHEA
University of West London
London, England

I

Global Health Nursing in Clinical Practice

Determined to Make a Difference

We begin this collection of narratives from the field with colleagues who describe their path to a career in global health. In doing so, they reflect the width and breadth of knowledge and practice that nursing offers to individuals and communities around the world. A great sense of purpose is conveyed in these narratives. The authors clearly demonstrate the importance of having solid clinical skills, which they bring to a variety of settings and populations. I appreciate the message they convey that we shouldn't just jump in because we want to. Instead, we need to be prepared and thoughtful as we approach our work.

1

An Unexpected Path

From Domestic Cancer Care to Global HIV Work

MARIE COLLINS DONAHUE

Editor's Note: Marie Donahue builds upon her U.S. experience in pediatric oncology to become involved with global AIDS work in Africa. She weaves experiences in the United States and Rwanda with others in Tanzania and Malawi to discuss the difficult decisions facing nurses and parents regarding the health and well-being of children.

TWO PLANETS

My initial desire to work with vulnerable children—those diagnosed with cancer—led me early in my career to Memorial Sloan-Kettering Cancer Center (MSKCC) in New York City. After several years of staff nursing, I felt the need to broaden my horizons and expand my scope of practice. I enrolled in a nurse practitioner program while continuing my work in oncology. While in graduate school, nearly all of my clinical placements were in some of the most impoverished communities in New York City and included immigrants, both documented and undocumented, from virtually every part of the world. Both settings—MSKCC and my graduate school clinical placements—served children from across the globe, but the similarity ended there. I was shocked by the glaring disparity in access to health care between the oncology patients I cared for at MSKCC and those in my clinical placements. I felt that I inhabited two planets.

On the first planet, the world-renowned midtown hospital with state-of-the-art equipment, children received unlimited medical resources—any and all diagnostic studies, chemotherapeutic regimens, surgical and radiological interventions, and when all else failed cutting-edge experimental treatments. In addition, children and their families received comprehensive psychosocial support, including access to psychologists and social workers; recreational therapy; a hospital-based school program; and gifts, parties, and access to free summer camps. No financial expense was spared for these children. Yet despite all these efforts, many of course died.

The other planet was a short distance away in Harlem and the Bronx. In this world, the only health care many children received was provided by nurse practitioner graduate students at school-based health clinics. Some of the conditions that our patients developed could have easily been prevented if they had had access to primary care services, and for just a fraction of the cost of treatment that my oncology patients received. This experience broadened my definition of "vulnerable" to include not just those children made fragile by disease processes but to those rendered defenseless because of socioeconomic status: in other words, the poor.

Despite the sometimes unfathomable distance between my two planets, there was an area of overlap, unknown to me at the time, but one that would foreshadow my global health work. At MSKCC, we were seeing infants on our unit with unusual opportunistic infections, such as *pneumocystis carinii* pneumonia, toxoplasmosis, and cytomegalovirus, along with failure to thrive and developmental delays. We also noticed that one or both of their parents appeared to be ill, often very thin and wasted. My friends who were working on adult units were caring for patients with what was then called "GRID" (an acronym for "gay-related immune deficiency"). At that time we knew very little about this condition.

During one of my clinical experiences in the emergency department (ED) of a Bronx hospital, I evaluated an 8-year-old boy who had shingles, an unusual diagnosis for a child. Given my work in oncology, my first suspicion was that he had become immunosuppressed from chemotherapy. His father told me that the boy's mother was being seen in the adult ED for pneumonia. When I presented his case to my preceptor, she started asking questions about the father and told me this child was in fact well known to her, and that both he and his parents had AIDS and were frequently seen in the emergency department (ED). She asked the father why he did not tell me that his child was HIV-infected; he replied, "She never asked me the question." Clearly, I had to learn to negotiate my way on this new planet, and learning to ask the right questions was just the start. Although

I initially thought this was the first HIV-infected child I ever took care of, I realized that those immunocompromised infants we had cared for were very likely HIV-infected as well.

As I learned the importance of the socio-ecological framework to health care, I became curious about the larger field of public health and I enrolled in the MPH program at Harvard University's School of Public Health. There I encountered the field of "International Health" (what we now call "global") and learned a great deal from international students enrolled there. Still, the possibility of working internationally did not yet occur to me.

PEDIATRIC HIV

After completing my MPH, I moved back to New York City and began working in a pediatric HIV program as both the research coordinator for perinatal and pediatric HIV clinical trials and as a nurse practitioner at a very large academic medical center. The field of HIV had come a long way in the 6 years since I saw my first "official" HIV-infected child. We learned that HIV was caused by a virus and knew how transmission occurred; we discovered how the virus operated to hijack the immune system and that the patterns of disease progression varied greatly between adults and children; and we had developed a laboratory test that would identify infected individuals as well as keep the blood supply safe. Zidovudine, a drug that had been used unsuccessfully for cancer treatment, was found to be effective in slowing HIV-AIDS disease progression.

But the most exciting development of all involved the pediatric population. Nearly all HIV-infected children acquired their infections from their mothers some time during pregnancy, delivery, or through breastfeeding. Just prior to my beginning work in the clinic, a landmark clinical trial had just been published that demonstrated that maternal-to-child transmission (MTCT) of HIV could be reduced by 66% with the use of zidovudine. This clinical trial was the beginning of one of the greatest public health success stories the world has ever known, and it led to the virtual elimination of pediatric HIV in the United States. Sadly, this public health achievement did not extend to the developing world. More than any other area on the globe, sub-Saharan Africa remained the disease epicenter: the virus raged there, and it remained virtually untouched by these astounding medical advances.

After 5 years, I moved to another pediatric HIV clinic in New York City. I wanted to work with one of the premier pediatric HIV physicians in the country who had cared for the earliest pediatric HIV patients. This was in 2004, when the world saw how devastating the HIV epidemic had become in Africa, yet people did not generally believe that treatment would be "practical" there. Many believed that Africans were simply too uneducated to understand treatment; that they lacked the ability to be adherent to any complex medication regimens; and that the lack of health care infrastructure simply prohibited treatment. Against such views, our clinic director helped develop a program at the Columbia University School of Public Health to show that HIV care and treatment *can* work in the developing world. This novel program was called MTCT-Plus (mother-to child transmission), and its goal was to provide care and treatment for pregnant HIV-infected women *and* their families (the latter indicated by the "Plus" in the program title). MTCT-Plus featured a family-centered, multidisciplinary model with teams of American HIV clinical experts deployed to several African countries to help organize clinics and teach local health care providers how to provide care and treatment for HIV-pregnant women and all members of their families. The program had been running for 1 year when I arrived at the clinic. By now I understood HIV clinical practice as well as the complicated psychosocial issues associated with HIV and was eager to share my knowledge with a new population. I believed that my skills as a nurse were especially valuable since over 90% of those providing health care in the developing world are nurses. I asked my clinical director to allow me to be part of the team traveling to Africa and she agreed. I had no idea this opportunity would lead to my working in global health for the next decade.

GLOBAL HEALTH

HIV Is the Least of Their Problems: Poverty in Tanzania

My entrée into global health was thus both a function of fate—being in the right place at the right time—as well as a logical next step in the trajectory of my aspiration to work with the underserved. My work was made possible by the convergence of two factors: a solid grounding in pediatric HIV care, and the announcement of the President's Emergency Plan for AIDS Relief (PEPFAR) by President George W. Bush in 2003. PEPFAR's initial mandate was broad and ambitious: to provide antiretroviral drugs to those HIV-infected in the developing world. As a result of its substantial funding, many nongovernmental organizations (NGOs) and universities expanded HIV programs already in operation (including MTCT-Plus), while others developed new programs to "scale-up" antiretroviral rollout.

Initially, MTCT-Plus was designed to provide didactic training sessions for local HIV health care providers. We quickly learned, however, that lectures alone would not be sufficient to equip these nurses, physicians, pharmacy staff, and mental health counselors for the management of complicated issues involved in HIV care. The program thus expanded to include clinical mentoring in the field. By getting out of the classroom and into clinics and hospitals, I began to understand how simply exporting our programs to the developing world would not guarantee successful outcomes and that solutions for the United States were not necessarily solutions in other parts of the world. I learned that HIV was often perceived as the least of the problems families faced, as unlikely as this might sound. Indeed, poverty, food insecurity, poor infrastructure, and lack of transportation rendered high-quality HIV care and treatment almost impossible at times.

One example from a clinic in rural Tanzania illustrates this fact. One of my first clinical mentoring experiences involved a mother who brought her 10-year-old son to the clinic. She carried him in her arms as if he were still an infant because he was unable to walk and had severe failure to thrive. He had been started on an antiretroviral regimen 1 month prior to the clinic visit, but for the past 3 weeks had developed severe diarrhea, likely due to lack of potable water. When I asked why she did not bring him to the clinic earlier, she said she had transportation money for just one visit per month and knew that if she came to the clinic when he first became ill she would miss the monthly visit to pick up his medications. I recommended to the clinical officer that we admit the child to the hospital and begin aggressively treating his dehydration and malnutrition. However, I learned that although the hospital could give the child IV fluids, it did not supply food or nutritional supplementation to any patient. This horrified me. I brought to this experience my naïve assumption that a resource as basic as food would be provided at a hospital. In my desperation to help, I gave the mother money to buy food for the child, but knew that it was not a sustainable solution to such an overwhelming problem. Part of me felt that I was giving her money to ease the guilt I felt about my own privilege.

While PEPFAR provided medication and the resources for basic HIV care, its mandate did not address the myriad concurrent conditions that exacerbated HIV. I began to think about Maslow's Hierarchy of Needs: without addressing the basics at the bottom of the pyramid—necessities such as food, clean water, and transportation—what good would our efforts ultimately achieve? The lack of focus on broader health determinants has been something I have struggled with in every resource-limited setting I have ever worked. Our work in global health too often focuses on treating complex disease processes, such as HIV and multidrug-resistant tuberculosis, while ignoring the fundamentals of health such as clean water and adequate sanitation. I am certainly not alone in my belief that if we addressed disease and health fundamentals simultaneously, much better outcomes would result overall. Nor am I the first to propose that solutions to common problems such as malnutrition are much simpler and cheaper than complicated antiretroviral regimens. As Paul Farmer once stated in a lecture I attended, "Last time I checked, we had a cure for malnutrition. It's called food." Global health problems should not be addressed vertically, so to speak, but integrated horizontally with efforts to improve economic conditions, infrastructure, and educational systems. I knew this in theory, but attempting to treat this young Tanzanian boy brought the message home to me in an unforgettable way.

Much of my global health experience up to this point had been with programs designed for short-term deployments in the field, lasting from 2 to 6 weeks. Despite some gains in education and clinical practice, I felt that these assignments were on the whole too short to provide sustainable progress. Over the past 10 years working in global health, my conviction regarding the importance of broadly conceived health factors has only deepened. A narrow focus on the delivery of antiretrovirals without addressing larger care issues such as stigma and providing psychosocial supports does not result in optimal outcomes. While expanding the focus remains crucial, I saw that an even more urgent problem was the critical shortage of a well-educated health care workforce in countries throughout sub-Saharan Africa. To address precisely this need, the United States Agency for International Development (USAID) began to develop programs to mobilize what is now known as "human resources for health."

Cultural Determinants of Care—Rwanda

One novel program aimed at improving the quality and quantity of the health care workforce was recently implemented in Rwanda. Unlike typical short-term projects, this program was designed to last 7 years with cadres of nurses, physicians, and health administrators deployed for at least 1 year each. Based in hospitals, nursing, and medical schools, the premise of the program was that the year-long commitment would provide an opportunity to work toward sustainable improvement. I was pleased to be chosen for the team. My years in global health work had taught me that it is important to understand broader aspects of culture—for example, political, economic, social, professional—prior to suggesting change. I decided that the first several weeks should be devoted to observation, so I could better understand the system and get to know my Rwandan colleagues. I believed strongly that it is critical to establish trust and build relationships, and now I had the luxury of time to do so. Or so I thought.

Baby Lea

When I first arrived at the hospital, the most critical patient on the ward was Lea, a 2.5-year-old child who had just tested positive for HIV. She was admitted with severe HIV-disease progression and had recently been effectively orphaned (her mother was likely either too sick to care for her or had herself died). Lea was so emaciated from her infection that she was the size of an average 8-month old. She was extremely developmentally delayed: she could not crawl, walk, or talk. Her muscle tone was so weak that she could not sit without support. She was so withdrawn that she would not make eye contact or even reach out to grab the small toys or lollipops that I offered her. I had seen children like her before and knew that if we intervened quickly to provide intensive nutritional support and HIV treatment she was likely to recover within just a few weeks. A standard plan of care indicated that the first priority was to treat her severe malnutrition; given its severity, she would require nasogastric tube (NGT) feedings with a specialized formula every 3 hours. Monitoring her response to the feedings did not require any high-tech equipment, but rather the simple use of a scale, a growth chart, and paper to document her intake and output. Once her hydration status was stabilized and she could tolerate feedings, an antiretroviral medication regimen to treat her HIV infection was to begin. This consisted of three medications that required administration every 12 hours. Strict adherence to this schedule was necessary to assure effectiveness as well as to prevent drug resistance.

The hospital had a protocol for treating children like Lea who were diagnosed with HIV. Medications were dispensed by the HIV clinic and left at the bedside for caregivers (such as, family or friends) to administer. Nurses did not provide medication teaching or oversight of the medications and knew very little about how the medications worked and even less about the side effects.

Although the nurses placed the feeding tube, they believed that the responsibility of administering the feeds and medications were the caregivers'. Lea's caregivers were several nuns who rotated from the orphanage she had come from. Their intentions were good; however, consistency of care—important to a child as fragile as Lea—was compromised.

Given the critical nature of Lea's condition, I decided to postpone my observation of the ward and to focus my efforts instead on educating the staff about how to optimize care for Lea. Surely once nurses were educated and supported, nursing care would improve. That, at least, was my assumption. I offered brief PowerPoint lectures on pediatric HIV, malnutrition, growth and development assessment of the child, and I included specific nursing care elements that were critical for Lea. There were no policies or procedures regarding NGT feedings, so I developed a brief guide to the practice. As there was no standard documentation record for intake and output, I developed a simple form designed to capture essential information including daily weight. I developed a schedule of feeding times and posted it above the bed.

Each day when I arrived on the ward, however, I noted that Lea's weight had not been checked. So I asked the nursing students on the ward to weigh Lea and record her weight in the patient record—but in vain. My concern and frustration grew. After several days, I concluded that I should model the behavior, so I weighed her and completed the documentation myself. Each morning, however, I noted that the feedings had not been recorded and realized that the nurses had not administered the feeds. After a week, I took the additional step of administering feeds myself, thinking again that modeling the behavior might be an effective approach. The program's philosophy was to mentor local health care providers, rather than to intervene directly in patient care. However, in this very urgent case, I decided that teaching by example was the best route.

On morning rounds, the physicians spoke about the importance of feedings and the nurses nodded in agreement. Their nod was gradually becoming familiar to me. It seemed to indicate acknowledgement of a superior's requests, but did not apparently reflect agreement or intent. The nurses' response was to report that some of the nuns were reluctant to administer the feedings. At times, Lea pulled out her feeding tube, which according to the nurses was an indication that Lea didn't like the tube. I reviewed techniques with them to prevent this from occurring (for example, wrapping her hands in gauze, distraction, and so on). Communication was clearly a problem. Most of the nurses I worked with did not speak English, and as I did not speak Kinyarwanda, I had little idea what they actually thought about my recommendations. Nor did I know what they thought Lea's basic problem was or what they thought should be done about it. In retrospect, I also had no real understanding of how the nurses defined their role and that of nursing in general.

Over 3 weeks, Lea's condition deteriorated. She did not gain weight and she actually developed a pressure ulcer over a protruding hip bone (in part likely due to her severe malnutrition and compromised immune function). Her cries became weaker; my exasperation grew. What else could I do, I wondered? Upon arriving in the ward on a Monday morning, Lea had become so severely dehydrated that she was in shock. Her extremities were cold, her cries barely audible. In reviewing her chart from the weekend, I noted that there was, once again, no documentation regarding feeding or fluids. My Rwandan partner reported that Lea had not received any feedings, as she had pulled out her NGT and it had not been replaced. Despite the lack of any oral intake, no attempts at providing intravenous fluids had been made. When I discussed this with my partner, she stated that there had only been one nurse on duty over the weekend and she was too overwhelmed to attend to the needs of all the patients. The census that weekend was just six, and the other five patients were stable. Lea was clearly the most critical patient. I was completely baffled as to why the nurse did not prioritize her efforts and care for the child who was most in need. And I wondered—as I still do—why the physician on duty that weekend had not intervened. That morning, the ward physician finally moved into action by starting an intravenous line and prescribing fluid boluses to correct her severe dehydration. But by then it was far too late.

Lea died the next morning, shortly before my arrival on the ward. Despite all that I had observed in the previous 3 weeks, I still felt alarm over her death and was outraged that a child could die of malnutrition and dehydration *while* being treated in a hospital equipped to help her. My Rwandan partner expressed sincere sorrow at her suffering ("poor Lea") and spoke about how she was in a much better place now. Her response was very telling, but to be honest I didn't fully understand it at the time. I tried to make sense of the case with my U.S. colleagues. One American nurse who had been a missionary in the country some 30 years earlier flatly told me "they don't value life the way that we do." Other colleagues talked about the "lack of motivation" of the nurses, asserting that "they just didn't care about their patients." These conclusions are seductively simplistic. They appear to explain the phenomenon of apparently conscious neglect—we would frankly call it malpractice—but they do so in a manner that is not only condescending and judgmental, but in a way that dodges the real enigma. What was going on? Though I thought of Lea as one of those "vulnerable children" I had always tried to serve, I was wrong to assume that the lived reality of Rwandan nurses was comparable to that of me or my U.S. colleagues.

Almost 8 months into my deployment, I met a Belgian nurse who had lived in several African countries for over 20 years. She is now a "cross-cultural coach" working with employees of large Western companies that have relocated to Africa. She provides counseling to employees and their families to help with the transition not just to Africa but also to life back home once their assignment is over. She helped me understand that in environments where there is little autonomy and few resources, it is common to accept the role that "fate" plays in life, and that this is actually an understandable survival strategy. After reflecting further on this case, I believe it is quite possible that the nurses caring for this very fragile child saw her immense suffering and decided—perhaps subconsciously—that by not intervening her suffering would end and she would be ushered into that "better place" my partner had spoken of. Rwanda is after all overwhelmingly Christian; the belief in a better afterlife may have made death a more acceptable "option," particularly in a country that had experienced such widespread death so recently. What would Lea's life have been like had she survived this hospitalization? Perhaps the nurses were factoring in some of these considerations as well. Maybe they saw the larger picture more clearly than I.

The Teacher Becomes the Student

After this incident, I realized that nursing practice on the pediatric ward bore little resemblance to my own nursing practice in America. It gradually dawned on me that my definition of nursing practice was not relevant in this situation and that I was the one who struggled to reconcile differences, not my African colleagues. I realized I had attended to discrete tasks rather than paying attention to the larger picture. I tried to go back to basics and reminded myself that the basic education of a nurse in Rwanda is equivalent to a high school diploma in the United States, and that "upgrading" the level of education was after all one of the *major* goals of our program, not something that could be presumed. I had to be mindful that it is not realistic or appropriate to expect the nurses to function as my colleagues and I do back home.

Another factor at work in the apparent miscommunication between the nurses and I regarding Lea's care is what one might call "NGO fatigue." Like many other developing countries, Rwanda has been inundated with NGOs from Western countries coming to do "good" work. The effect of this well-intended foreign input is not always as sanguine as we might like to believe. At the end of my year, for example, the Director of Nursing revealed the following to me:

> We have had so many white people come in here and tell us what to do. They were arrogant and rude and did not respect us or support us.... They were very hard to work with and many nurses had to take sick leave because they were so stressed from the work. When I heard you were coming, I said, "Oh no, what will these people do to us."

Finally, the life circumstances of nurses with whom I worked certainly play a significant role in their ability to work effectively. These circumstances also affect the desire and energy they are able to marshal toward making changes in their settings. I learned that many nurses have inadequate access to food and that the modest meal that is provided at my hospital may be the only meal of the day for them. I know that many hold second jobs, in addition to the 50 hours they are scheduled to work at the hospital, just in order to make ends meet for their families. As if that weren't enough, many are caring for sick and elderly parents in addition to their own children. Nurses sometimes experience salary reductions when the government experiences budget shortfalls. Many of these nurses are the primary breadwinners for their families. I have also heard stories of the struggles many nurses have faced in the aftermath of the genocide—unimaginable personal losses and deprivation during their childhoods, with few mental health services available to help them cope. How does one even begin to measure these factors?

Expanding the Circle: HIV Care in Malawi

My experience with baby Lea echoes in many respects a qualitative research study I led in Malawi some years before (Donahue, Dube, Sheehan, Umar, & Van Rie, 2012). At the time, I was not able to map one experience on to the other. There are, I was to learn, additional factors that impede a simple "transfer" of Western care to local populations.

In Malawi, high-quality HIV programs had become available specifically for care and treatment of early infant HIV infection, but acceptance of such programs remained low. I wanted to explore possible cultural norms that guided the decisions HIV-infected women made regarding how they sought care for their babies. Many factors seemed obvious; for example, disclosure to the partner, stigma, gender inequality, lack of autonomy, and economic barriers. But what initially seems obvious is rarely the whole answer.

So what did we learn? Surprisingly, the study revealed that disclosure was not a factor. Virtually all women in the study had disclosed their HIV status to their partners (although many had not disclosed to other family members and few had disclosed to their friends or neighbors). Second, I discovered that maternal "autonomy" was a positive factor to an extent I had not thought possible in a traditional, patriarchal society. Although women noted that their male partners were formally the decision makers in the family, they reported that even if their husbands disagreed about the need for testing, they could seek it for their babies without fear of reprisal.

Further, we discovered that the concept of autonomy extends to health care providers who are viewed as key authority figures. Women tended to believe that if they followed what the doctor or nurse advised their babies would be healthy. This thinking did not take into account the fact that following recommendations does not guarantee positive outcomes for their babies and thus may ultimately undermine the confidence women have in treatment recommendations. In addition, following some of the recommendations was often not practical for women, as they might arouse suspicion of HIV infection by other family members.

We also found that because many women did not believe they could disagree with or question their providers, they were often confused about medication and testing recommendations. Furthermore, health care providers themselves were accustomed to practicing as authority figures and their methods of practice initially did not include an engaging style. These findings were enlightening, reminding me once again of the danger of importing and imposing Western assumptions. But one additional finding was of particular note—and still defies full explanation.

"Letting" Children Die

While many of our questions asked about stigma, disclosure, and beliefs about the effectiveness of treatment, one asked directly why some women did not bring their babies in for testing even though treatment was available. Several mothers told us that some might allow their sick babies to die and in some cases might even use poison to hasten their deaths. Why would mothers let their children die? Although our interviewer training included techniques in how to further probe responses, *none* of the interviewers explored this theme with participants, very likely because of the highly charged nature of the response. I struggled mightily with this finding. Because the response was not limited to just one mother, I felt it was critical to address it in the data analysis. I hesitated because I feared that my background—a White Westerner who had spent only 6 weeks in the country—might lead me to portray the study participants in a reckless, uninformed manner.

I found help in the work of anthropologist Nancy Scheper-Hughes (1992). In her ethnographic work with women living in Brazilian shantytowns, she reveals how the high expectancy of child death is a powerful shaper of maternal thinking and practice. She posits that day-to-day moral thinking is guided by a variation of "lifeboat ethics," which basically asks who should be saved (and who not) when it is impossible to save all. Yet another anthropologist, Sarah Hrdy (1999), describes infant abandonment and infanticide as a continuum that has existed throughout history. She observes that mothers do not set out to harm their infants. She believes that maternal behavior cannot be properly evaluated in isolation from the mothers' particular socioeconomic circumstances. While Malawi and Brazil are on opposite sides of the globe and have very different cultures, they share the characteristic of extreme poverty and high child mortality rates. Although I could not assume that the Brazilian experience was the equivalent of the Malawian one, I had found a perspective that would allow for more nuanced exploration. Those Malawian mothers who did not bring their HIV-infected children to clinic for free care may have been making a decision not against life, but *for* the lives of their other children and dependents.

LESSONS LEARNED?

As I learned in the cases of baby Lea and of those Malawian children "allowed" to die, we cannot focus exclusively on the individual patient to the exclusion of the broader social setting. Maybe we simply don't want to accept the fact that the rock-bottom premise of "life boat ethics" really is true after all—such as, that not all people can be saved. Not in the short run at least. Perhaps we focus on the alleged "malpractice" of individuals to avoid looking at that larger tragedy in which survival really is sometimes a zero-sum game. This may not be a very optimistic or "American" point of view, but it is one I am struggling to understand to this day.

Finally, as I learned during my year abroad in Africa, while it may be terribly important to go on a long "listening tour" before introducing changes in clinical practice, I cannot pretend that I simply want to understand what I see or hear. If we are honest—if I am honest—we want to *change* some aspects of what is seen or heard as well. I have never, since the beginning of my nursing career, been a disinterested, dispassionate observer of the suffering of vulnerable children. The dilemma in global health is about developing strategies so we have the insight to respect and understand the lives of others and in doing so to work with them, to bring change and relief.

REFERENCES

Donahue, M. C., Dube, Q., Sheehan, A. D., Umar, E., & Van Rie, A. (2012). "They have already thrown away their chicken": Barriers affecting participation by HIV-infected women in care and treatment programs for their infants in Blantyre, Malawi. *AIDS Care: Psychological and Socio-medical Aspects of AIDS/HIV, 24*(10), 1233–1239.

Hrdy, S. B. (1999). *Mother nature: A history of mothers, infants, and natural selection*. New York, NY: Pantheon.

Scheper-Hughes, N. (1992). *Death without weeping: The violence of everyday life in Brazil*. Berkeley, CA: University of California Press.

2

Patience, Understanding, and Advocacy

Scrubbing Babies in Africa

TINA ANSELMI-MOULAYE

Editor's Note: Tina Anselmi-Moulaye describes her journey from being a young Peace Corps volunteer to becoming a nurse-midwife who transfers skills honed while working with at-risk populations in the United States to vulnerable populations abroad. Like Marie Donahue (Chapter 1), Tina accepts a position in Rwanda to provide training to midwives. Although she speaks French fluently, Tina encounters communication problems, which she seeks to ameliorate with caring and insight.

I always knew I would become a Peace Corps Volunteer. I have a vivid childhood memory of watching the Peace Corps television advertisement where a man stood in an African village digging a well and the voice said, "It's the toughest job you'll ever love." I was 9 or 10 years old when I saw that commercial and I knew that traveling to faraway places and meeting interesting people was something I wanted to do.

I grew up in a small town in Wyoming, and I caught the travel bug early. I traveled to the south of France as an exchange student in high school. I loved everything about France: the food, the wine and cheeses, the language, and my host family. So in college, I returned to study for a semester in Aix-en-Provence, and pursued a bachelor's degree in French teaching. But there was one small problem. After graduating with a degree in French teaching, I realized that I didn't want to be a French teacher. I wanted to travel.

After college, I visited a close Peace Corps friend in Ecuador. She was a health volunteer and I was able to accompany her to several rural health clinics. My friend noticed that I always gravitated toward the pregnant women—listening to and sitting with them. The more time I spent in clinics and reading about women's health, the more I wanted to learn. What were the struggles and health problems that accompanied pregnancy? How could I help improve the health of women and children? That trip to Ecuador reinforced my desire to become a midwife and to join the Peace Corps.

When I applied to the Peace Corps, my goal was to spend as much time on labor wards as possible in order to make a final decision. Did I want to become a midwife? Could I really help women give birth? Could I tolerate the suffering and all the blood and bodily fluids that come with the birthing process? I wasn't sure about anything, but I was eager to put myself to the test.

PEACE CORPS—MALI

The Peace Corps sent me to Mali in West Africa. Like my friend in Ecuador, I worked as a health volunteer. I gave presentations to parents who came to vaccinate their children about malaria prevention, nutrition, rehydration, and family planning.

My work was enjoyable because I was able to observe the nurses and midwives. Their interactions with each other and their patients were fascinating to me. At times, the midwife helped me measure the height of the uterus and listen to the baby's heartbeat. I was quickly falling in love with the art of midwifery, as well as the people I worked with.

In the maternity unit, I was able to observe care given to mothers. The midwives gave me the job of bathing the newborn babies. They instructed me to scrub the babies vigorously in order to remove all the secretions and vernix (the thick, white, waxy substance that often covers a newborn at birth). The midwives told me that if I didn't clean the baby well enough, he would smell bad for the rest of his life. So you can be sure I scrubbed and cleaned the babies very well! The babies were often born very limp and slightly blue, but by the time I finished scrubbing, they were crying at the top of their lungs. I was having the time of my life and I knew, without a doubt, that I wanted to become a midwife.

I now realize that by scrubbing the newborn babies, I was actually stimulating the baby to breath and cry. When newborn babies are having trouble transitioning to external life, they often look limp and blue and need help taking that first breath. Stimulation, or rubbing and drying the baby and keeping the baby warm are the best ways to help these babies breath. Thank goodness this "cleaning" was performed at each birth in Mali, because without this stimulation many babies might not have survived.

My time in the Peace Corps taught me a lot about life and death and delivering babies. When it was time to leave, I was sad, but I knew I wasn't saying goodbye. I knew I would return to Africa.

NURSING SCHOOL—BALTIMORE

I returned home intent on laying the groundwork to become a midwife. I completed an accelerated nursing program at Johns Hopkins University. I practiced in an emergency department for 2 years while also working part-time at a birthing center, which gave me a chance to continue learning about birth. I then returned to school to get my master's degree in nursing-midwifery. The year I started graduate school was monumental for another reason because my boyfriend and I decided to get married. I met my husband in Baltimore through mutual friends but he also happened to be from Mali. He is from Timbuktu.

MIDWIFERY—EL PASO

After graduation, we moved to El Paso, Texas where I worked with the National Health Service Corps in order to help pay off student loans. I worked for 2 years as a nurse-midwife in a clinic run by Catholic nuns on the border between Texas and Mexico.

Claudia

My first experience working with a mother who had a fetal demise was in El Paso. I will call this mother Claudia. I got the phone call from Claudia's husband saying that she was having contractions and they were getting stronger. After asking several questions to assess the situation, I suggested she come to the clinic for a labor check. I remembered the most important question at the last moment and so before the husband hung up, I shouted, "Excuse me, is the baby moving well?" There was a conversation between the two and when he came back to the phone he said, "No, she says she hasn't felt the baby move since last night." My heart sank and I told her to go to the hospital right away.

To my surprise, a couple of hours later Claudia and her husband arrived at the clinic. I asked them how she was feeling and why they had not gone to the hospital. Her reply, although not unexpected, was what I had feared. She was worried about being deported if she went to the hospital. So she didn't go. I quickly put her in a room and began to listen for a fetal heart beat. I heard nothing. I got the sonogram machine and searched for cardiac movement in the baby's chest. I saw no movement. I had to explain to Claudia and her husband that I could not hear the baby's heartbeat.

It was tragic to experience this loss with the family. My heart broke for them. It was also tragic for me to imagine that if she hadn't been afraid of deportation, Claudia would have gone straight to the hospital, where it might have been possible to save her baby.

I'm sure that if you ask any midwife or obstetrician to recall the first fetal demise, he or she will recount all the details. It is a very difficult rite of passage. I couldn't help but worry that I had done something wrong. It took time to process what had happened and to recover. I often think about Claudia and I send her my thoughts and prayers. The memory of her loss is why I am so motivated to educate women and mothers. If I can do anything, on any level to prevent these losses, I will do it.

When my contract in El Paso ended, my family and I moved back to Baltimore. My husband and I thought about moving back to Mali, but because we had two young sons we decided to stay in the United States for a few more years. I got a job working as a nurse-midwife in a busy hospital that had over 4,000 births a year. The job was different than the one in El Paso. I functioned more like a medical resident, which allowed me to assist in cesarean sections and to manage most high-risk complications in pregnancy.

I also became a clinical instructor for nursing students during their rotation on labor & delivery and postpartum. I enjoyed teaching nursing students because they were seeing births for the first time and motivated to learn as much as possible. Teaching is not like clinical practice. It requires a different type of patience and objectivity. Students learn differently and you have to constantly assess their progress in order to support their learning. It is a balancing act between constructive criticism and motivation. It is challenging on many levels, but important work.

MENTOR—RWANDA

When I first heard about the Midwifery Mentor job, I was skeptical. In the world of international development, it is difficult to find employment in a setting where you can provide clinical services. Generally, the only way to work in a hospital overseas is as a volunteer. There are paid jobs working with governmental or nongovernmental organizations, but most are on a consulting level or entail a lot of paperwork like applying for grants and writing reports.

I am happy to report that the international community is beginning to fund projects where health professionals work with their counterparts in health centers and hospitals in developing nations. My job in Rwanda was one of those jobs. I was assigned to work as a Midwifery Mentor in a maternity unit in one of the referral hospitals in the capital city of Kigali. My job was to train midwifery staff and students working in the maternity unit. I was thrilled.

I spent the first few weeks with the midwives observing their practices. We were told in orientation that it was important to spend some time observing before making any changes. This was difficult to do, but because of my Peace Corps experience, I knew it was necessary in order to earn the trust of my colleagues. Obviously, my work as a mentor was different than my work as a Peace Corps Volunteer. I now possessed the skills to help improve midwifery practice and so it was more difficult not to jump in and do the work. I did jump in in emergency situations when lives were at risk, but in general, I tried to observe practices and build relationships in the first few weeks.

The first challenge I encountered was regarding my role in the hospital. The local midwives were often confused as to why I wasn't taking a patient assignment. They told me on several occasions, "Learning is done in the classroom, but in the hospital, you work. Why are you trying to teach in the hospital? If you want to help us you need to start taking care of patients."

Development work requires that you constantly ask yourself "will this work continue after I am gone?" If the response is no, you must take a different approach. For instance, if I had taken a patient assignment, as the midwives requested, when I left there would be one less midwife and patient care would suffer. However, if I stand next to the midwives and students and help them improve their skills by asking questions and demonstrating assessments and interventions, the whole system improves and is stronger. If I can demonstrate effective mentoring, the midwives will develop effective mentoring skills themselves. This encourages teaching and, hopefully, improvements to continue.

Nursing and midwifery in a Rwandan hospital is very different than in the United States, which is another reason why my taking a patient assignment would not have been a good idea. In the United States, hospitals are fully stocked and sterile instruments are always available. You always have the instruments you need and probably have the best product on the market available to perform your job. The work environment is also team-oriented. I was used to working in a health care system that ran like a well-oiled machine. You could trust that every team member would do his or her job and, therefore, you could easily perform your job safely and successfully. The reality in Rwanda was far different from what I was used to.

One morning a midwife asked for my help. She said that she was having trouble breaking the bag of water for a patient who was being induced. She asked if I would try. I got a full history on the patient including the position of the baby's head, because if it is not down enough into the pelvis, the umbilical cord can slide out with the rushing water, causing a cord prolapse. A cord prolapse is an obstetrical emergency and it is important to avoid this at all costs.

The report sounded like an appropriate clinical situation, so I agreed to break the woman's water. I then spoke with the woman and explained what I was going to do and asked her permission. After she consented to the procedure, I asked for gloves. It is important to use sterile gloves to avoid infection. However, in this case, there were no sterile gloves and I was told they wash the gloves with an antiseptic before procedures such as this. I donned the gloves and the antiseptic solution was poured over my gloves onto the floor. When I put my hand out to ask for the amnihook (the small hook-shaped instrument used to break the bag of water), something strange happened. Instead of being given an amnihook, the midwife placed three cotton balls in my hand. We exchanged looks of confusion. I was wondering what I was supposed to do with three cotton balls and I'm sure the midwife wondered why I didn't know what to do with them. After a moment of silence, I asked what to do with the cotton balls. The midwife explained to me that I needed to clean the mother's perineum with the antiseptic solution before I began the exam. Okay, that made sense, so I cleaned the mother as I was told. I then performed a cervical exam to verify the cervical dilatation, effacement, and position of the baby's head. Once again I held out my hand to ask for the amnihook and I was given an object that looked like a miniature sword. Once again, I was quite puzzled. In the United States, the instrument we use is shaped like a croquet hook and we hook the bag of water to gently break it. We pull the bag away from the baby's head to avoid harming the baby. With a sword-like object, all I could do was poke forward toward the baby's head, which I was not comfortable doing. I hesitantly poked at the bag of fluid, gently scraping it in an attempt to break it. My efforts were not successful. I learned a valuable lesson that day; I was definitely not the expert in this maternity unit!

I learned, in fact, that it was best for me to sit back and observe so that I understood their working conditions and practices. I also needed to assess their level of midwifery knowledge and skill, which was lower than I expected. While observing the midwives, I had also noticed that little, if any, midwifery documentation existed in the patient charts. I decided to start my teaching by addressing the lack of documentation. I reasoned that I could touch on a variety of topics while discussing the importance of documenting patient care. For example, if I asked a midwife who was caring for a patient after a postpartum hemorrhage, "Why it is important that blood pressure be taken and documented on this patient?" Her response would help me assess her level of critical thinking. In this case, the midwife responded that she wasn't sure why taking blood pressure was important, but because the doctor ordered it, she must do it. I began to realize that the midwives were taught skills but no critical thinking. They were simply performing tasks that had been ordered by a physician but had little knowledge regarding assessment and monitoring of patients.

One day, while teaching vital signs skills and assessments, I learned that midwives were told that only doctors could use stethoscopes. As I explained that a stethoscope is absolutely used by midwives and nurses to assess cardiac and lung function, they looked at me with excitement. "You will teach us how to listen to a heart with a stethoscope?" When I said yes, they were like children learning how to ride a bike—nervous, but excited. One midwife put the stethoscope around her neck and began to strut through the room saying, "Look at me, I'm a doctor." The other midwives laughed uncontrollably.

To make things more confusing, I discovered that the midwives kept a list of completed tasks in a notebook. They used the notebook to communicate with the on-coming midwife in place of documenting in the patient chart. So as I addressed the importance of appropriate documentation, in general, I also tried to encourage use of the patient chart, rather than the notebook. In the end, the maternity unit managers decided to do away with the notebooks and instructed the midwives to refer to their notes in the patient chart when giving a verbal report each morning. It was gratifying to witness such a perfect example of how change can happen. I had pointed out something that needed improvement and the midwives, themselves, came up with the solution. Because they own the solution they are more likely to continue following their new protocol after I leave.

My advice to anyone wanting to work in international development is to have patience and accept small steps. Because health systems are often dysfunctional and practice standards are low, it is easy to become frustrated. I had been in Kigali for 4 months and it felt as if our only accomplishment was to have a shift report written in the patient chart instead of the notebook.

I had to remind myself that you can't compare nursing and midwifery in the United States with nursing and midwifery in Africa. It's like comparing apples and oranges. In fact, you shouldn't have any expectations about what you will find, because they will usually be wrong. You must go in with an open mind, ears, and eyes. If you have your own agenda, you will miss essential pieces of the puzzle and leave behind more problems than solutions.

Angel

I will share another story to illustrate clinical practices that needed to be addressed. A young woman was in labor with her first baby. I will call her Angel. She was giving birth without pain medication, as is true of all women in this hospital. The fetal heart tones had been within normal limits during her entire labor. She soon began to bear down with each contraction, indicating that she was probably fully dilated. Upon exam, she was, in fact, fully dilated with the baby's head almost visible.

When a woman becomes fully dilated, she is moved from a labor bed to a delivery bed. This means that she must get up and walk across the room to climb up onto a delivery table. All the while, her body is bearing down trying to push out a baby. Being a strong African woman, Angel walked across the room without complaining and got onto the delivery table. She then began to push with her contractions. After 30 minutes of pushing, Angel was not making enough progress to satisfy the Rwandan midwives. We listened to the baby's heart rate at the end of each contraction and noted that all was well. I was happy with the progress and status of the delivery, although I began to notice that everyone kept saying, "it's been too long, it's been 30 minutes" as they looked at each other with worry. One of the midwives stepped in to start oxytocin because she felt it was time to get the baby out. I calmly explained that the mother and baby were doing well. I told them not to start oxytocin.

Angel continued pushing without oxytocin and the fetal heart beat remained normal. Within a few minutes, a physician arrived asking what was happening. One of the midwives wanted to perform an episiotomy in order to get the baby out more quickly. I told her that it was too soon to cut an episiotomy and that everything was OK with the baby and the mother. I had to stop them from intervening on several occasions. Thank goodness no one tried to jump on the mother's abdomen to do fundal pressure (pushing downward on the top of the uterus), which was often done when they thought the baby needed to come out urgently. I had been involved in several situations where midwives cut episiotomies, gave rapid infusions of oxytocin, and applied fundal pressure in order to deliver a baby in haste. These are dangerous practices that result in babies being born in severe distress. I wasn't going to let that happen on my watch.

After an hour of pushing, Angel delivered a screaming, healthy baby boy. Apgar scores were 9 and 9, which is a perfect score. The fact that the baby was born healthy and the mother had no complications was a huge success story.

That evening, I reviewed the birth in my mind, wondering how I could use Angel's story as a teachable moment. I marked a few pages in my textbook on the second stage of labor (such as, the pushing part of labor) and prepared to discuss the birth with the midwives.

The following morning, we talked about the birth and why it was harmful to intervene with the natural progression of pushing. During the conversation, I learned the midwives were taught that when a mother pushes for more than 30 minutes the baby will be in distress. Because of the distress, it is necessary to get the baby out quickly. That was the reason for the panic and harmful fundal pressure. When I told them that it is normal for mothers to push for 2 hours as long as the baby's heartbeat patterns are good, they responded with looks of disbelief. One of the midwives said that in Africa things are different and when they push the babies are in distress. Another midwife stated, "But Tina we notice that whenever a baby is born after 30 minutes of pushing, the babies are always very sick. This proves to us that the babies are in distress after the mother pushes for 30 minutes."

I thought about this statement for a minute and then replied, "But it is the panic and harmful practices like fundal pressure that cause the baby to be sick, *not* the fact that the mother has been pushing for 30 minutes." What followed was silence as they thought about what I had said.

One of the managing midwives broke the silence by adding, "Yes, Tina wouldn't let me start oxytocin or do fundal pressure because the baby's heart rate was good. Then after an hour of pushing, the baby was born crying."

Having a trusted member of their management team support my statements encouraged the staff to trust what I was saying. We had an honest and open discussion about the case and I think we all learned something that morning. I learned their reasoning behind the harmful practices and the staff learned about fetal monitoring and which practices are harmful during pushing. I could tell we had had a breakthrough on two levels. First of all, I now knew that the midwives trusted me enough to talk honestly. They weren't telling me what they thought I wanted to hear and because of this, finally, the real learning could begin. Second, I now understood their point of view. Once I understood the "why" behind their actions, I could better explain the potential harm and how to do things differently. It was a good day for all of us.

Peace

Working in international development can be an emotional roller coaster. One day you feel you are finally making progress, and the next day you experience a setback. Keep in mind that setbacks are normal. We certainly have our share of them in the United States. I will share another story. I had developed a close friendship with one of my colleagues who worked as a supervisor in the maternity unit. I will call her Peace. Peace and I became friends almost immediately because she had a warm personality and we seemed to see eye to eye on many of the social issues surrounding the patients. Whenever I had a question, I went to Peace because I knew she could explain it in a way that I would understand. Because Peace and I were so close, she was honest with me when my behavior or questions seemed inappropriate. She would tell me why my actions were being taken the wrong way and how I could ask a question or approach a situation differently. I will forever be grateful for her friendship and guidance.

One afternoon Peace and I were working on a protocol regarding the administration of oxytocin. In obstetrics, oxytocin is used to stimulate or increase the force of uterine contractions. It is a common drug given in maternity units all over the world. Using it incorrectly can be very harmful to the laboring mother and also to the baby.

The oxytocin protocol was turning into a complex and lengthy document as I asked her to describe current practices related to the drug. I could tell she was getting restless, but I didn't know why. I pressed on because I felt we were on the verge of real progress. Finally, Peace couldn't hold her tongue any longer. It was obvious she was very frustrated. I will never forget the words she blurted out to me "*Tu sais, Tina, on veux que tu viens ici pour travailler avec nous, pour nous aider mais on ne veux pas que tu changes* tout!" "You know, Tina, we want you to come and work with us so you can help us, but we don't want you to change *everything*!"

I went to lunch with some other American nurses working at my hospital and told the story of what had just happened. I felt so frustrated and irritated. What was I doing wrong? What if I couldn't make any changes in that maternity unit and mothers and babies just kept dying? If Peace knows they need to change their practices, why does she become frustrated when we discuss how to implement those changes? I asked for advice from my family and friends and colleagues from all over the globe. Most people said that I just needed to be patient, that change takes time. Then one of my friends, a nurse, reminded me of how much resistance there is to small changes in the States. I began to realize that although the changes seemed small to me, to Peace and the other midwives, they were huge and threatened the foundation upon which they worked. I was asking for a lot of progress in a very short amount of time.

My work in Rwanda was part of a larger strategy in which other nurses will pick up where I left off. In time and with strong support of governmental and nongovernmental organizations and the nurses and midwives who represent the core of health services delivery, I am confident that the standards of care for women and children in Rwanda will improve.

I currently live in Qatar, but my future plans include more work in Africa. That is where my heart is. For now, I want to seize every opportunity that presents itself to me. I consider myself a lifelong learner, and each experience helps me become a more knowledgeable, qualified, and effective leader in global nursing.

I feel very strongly that we need to do a better job of marketing midwifery globally. Even though the Internet provides valuable information, I find that many people don't understand the amazing work we do. Writing books, creating websites or Facebook pages, and making documentaries is a good place to start. But I think we need to take it further. My dream is to be part of a global program of education regarding the work of midwives.

MY SOAPBOX

Please Be an Advocate for Nursing and Midwifery in Global Health!

I believe that developing nations need nursing and midwifery mentors more than physician mentors. The two professions represent two separate sets of skills. Although improvements in the skill set of physicians are needed, at this point in time, improving nursing skills should be the priority.

There are misconceptions about the capabilities and independence of work that is performed by nurses and midwives. The first misconception is that if you put a lot of emphasis on improving the quality of care provided by physicians the quality of nursing care will automatically raise as a consequence. The reality is, in fact, the exact opposite. To focus resources solely on physicians creates a system where the gap between the nurses and doctors grows—which results in communication and relationships becoming more disjointed. It is not a new finding that when communication is poor, health care outcomes are poor as well.

Another misconception is that nurses only do work that is ordered by the physician. Well-trained nurses and midwives have always served as primary care givers. Physicians arrive on the hospital unit to assess the patient and make medical decisions about the plan of care. He or she may spend 10 to 15 minutes reviewing a chart or assessing a patient and then writing a few new orders. The rest of the 24 hours of patient care is the nurse's responsibility. Continually monitoring the patient for health changes, medication administration, documentation, daily hygiene, getting to the toilet, answering questions about diseases, and translating what the doctor says into laymen terms are all duties of the nurse. And these are just the tip of the iceberg. Why would anyone think that what the physician does is more important than what a nurse does? If a doctor orders an antibiotic and the nurse gives it incorrectly or doesn't give it at all, the health of the patient is greatly compromised. The two jobs are different, but certainly, one is not more important or easier than the other.

If you create a system where improving the quality of nursing care is the priority, you will narrow the gap between doctors and nurses and create a team. You will improve the entire health care system from the ground up. If we focus on improving the assessment and monitoring of patients for the other 23 hours of the day, imagine how much we could improve patient outcomes. Working as a team improves outcomes. If you have nurses and midwives who question orders and who are allowed to use stethoscopes to assess patients and think independently within their scope of practice, you get great results. If you don't concentrate on improving nursing skills, the medical care may become more sophisticated while the nurses still don't know how to administer medications correctly or educate or assess patients. The system doesn't change. Nursing and midwifery education need to be priorities in global health care.

Whether we scrub babies in Mali or teach about stethoscopes in Rwanda, we each need to find a way to help improve global health care. We need qualified, motivated nurses and midwives to join the workforce!

3

A Worthy Endeavor

A Very Determined Nurse Achieves Her Goal

NAOMI J. BLACKMAN-ABDELLAOUI

Editor's Note: We follow Naomi Blackman-Abdellaoui's narrative as she describes her great determination to develop the skills required to work as a field nurse with Médecins Sans Frontières (MSF). In doing so, Naomi engaged in short-term global experiences, studied French, and partnered with her hospital administration to enhance her clinical and leadership skills. We share her sense of accomplishment as she reflects upon her first MSF mission. Her discussion regarding the suffering she witnessed while on mission is powerful.

No matter how hard I try, I cannot adequately articulate the depth or complexity of what I've witnessed while working in emergency humanitarian aid missions abroad. Furthermore, I cannot begin to tell the stories of all the people who are helping the most vulnerable and desperate populations at this very moment. What I can do is share my story as a nurse, with the hope that someone else will be inspired to help others in desperate need.

My path to global health began as an undergraduate student studying biology. In one class, we discussed Africa and the complexities of political corruption and its effect on everyday life. Clearly I had never thought about the politics of Africa. Throughout the discussion, students didn't speak about one country or one specific problem, they talked about the continent of Africa as if it were a small state or one country. Needless to say, many generalizations were made. I remember one student saying, "Why don't we just go over there and fix it?" Thankfully our professor quickly inserted herself into the dialogue, to help us understand that the complexities of the continent of Africa could not be easily "fixed" as my classmate suggested.

The student's statement stayed with me, because it made me curious to know more about international politics, access to health care, and global involvement in developing nations, especially in Africa. It also made me eager to learn more about other cultures and to see the world for myself.

NURSING SCHOOL

I used my biology degree to work for a biopharmaceutical company conducting fungicide research on soil samples, and then I transferred to a large pharmaceutical company where I was involved with pharmaceutical compound management. I applied to nursing school with the hope of fulfilling my desire to do more for other people and better understand the health care situation.

I enrolled in the nursing program at the University of North Carolina at Chapel Hill. Once I accepted the reality that I would have to eat, breathe, and sleep "nursing" in order to obtain a degree, I was able to focus on my goal of becoming a nurse. However, it was not until I started taking the community health nursing course that I realized I had a path toward working with vulnerable populations in the local community as well as in developing nations.

FIRST STEPS

The community health class offered a spring break trip to Guatemala for any student interested in learning about nursing and health care services in a developing nation. Despite my seriously tight budget, I found the means to get a passport and make this trip part of my nursing school experience. The time I spent in Guatemala lit a fire under my motivation to work in global health. I thought I had seen a lot of poverty while assessing the homeless population in my community, but I was surprised and troubled by the poverty I saw while visiting Guatemala. I had never seen street children begging for money or a war veteran, with missing limbs, leaned up against a building with a metal tin on the ground for collecting money. I had never been to a facility for the physically or mentally challenged where the staff did the best they could with almost nonexistent resources. Nor had I ever met a lay midwife who worked under difficult conditions to assist with home deliveries. Little did I know that this area of Guatemala (Antigua), though impoverished, had significantly more resources than most places I have visited since that first eye-opening voyage.

After the Guatemalan experience, I set my sights on going to Africa. I got a loan and booked a volunteer trip with International Service Learning (ISL) to commence 2 months after graduation from nursing school and 1 week after the NCLEX exam. My first experience as a new nurse was in rural Tanzania where I performed community health assessments and helped a national staff doctor manage the pharmacy during mobile clinics. I was the only licensed professional in the group; the others were undergraduate health science students. The local doctors spent time speaking with me about the differences in health care infrastructure in the United States compared with what I was seeing in rural Tanzania. They also asked if I had financial connections to fund their work, which unfortunately I did not have at the time.

What I observed, aside from a majestically green country filled with untouched nature, exotic animals seen on safari, and the beautiful smiles of kind children, were extremely hard-working medical professionals trying to manage major health needs grounded in intense poverty. I traveled with other volunteers to several villages where we conducted community health assessments, visited orphanages, and toured small clinics. I saw many orphans who had been abandoned by family due to their albinism (often associated with witchcraft) or HIV/AIDS status. During the community assessments and mobile clinics, we found many cases of malaria, tuberculosis, respiratory infections, diarrhea, and suspected HIV/AIDS. We were able to give some medications and make several referrals, but it felt as if we were doing too little too late and simply scratching the surface of what was needed. I was shocked by what I saw during my time in Tanzania and the effect on my life was profound. All I could think about was returning to do something more beneficial for populations in need.

Upon my return to North Carolina, I remember experiencing a bit of culture shock. My ideas about poverty, access to care, access to pharmaceuticals, vulnerable populations, electricity, water, and above all my responsibilities as a health care provider were challenged. I started looking for a nongovernmental organization (NGO) where I could work with seasoned health care providers—not students or

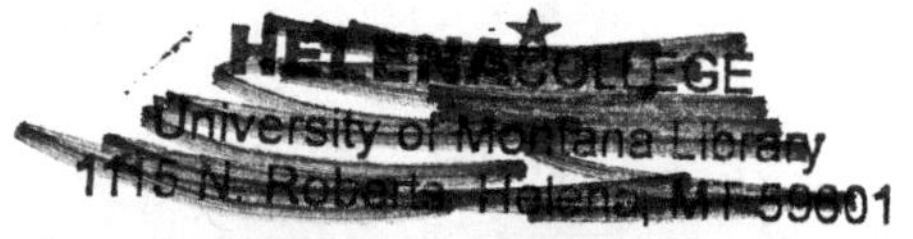

new graduates like myself—to provide assistance for communities with the greatest needs. I found what I considered to be the rock star of them all: Doctors without Borders, or Médecins Sans Frontières (MSF) as it known internationally—this was an organization that had won the Nobel Peace Prize. I had certainly heard of Doctors without Borders, but I had not closely followed their activities. After many visits to their website, I realized I was in way over my head and that I had a lot of work to do before I could even contemplate applying. After reading many country profiles and about MSF activity in those countries, it also became quite clear that I knew almost nothing about what was happening on the continent of Africa with respect to medical needs and access to health care, even though I had just come back from a 3-week trip to Tanzania.

TWO YEARS, THREE MONTHS, AND A LOT OF PREPARATION!

In order to prepare myself to apply for a position with MSF, I first had to learn how to be a "real" nurse. That meant having a minimum of 2 years of experience. Once I started working, I realized there was a mountain of nursing and critical thinking skills I had to master before I could move to the next level: training others and working as a charge nurse, which are two skills required by MSF. Work on a postsurgical step-down trauma/transplant unit at a top ranking hospital (Duke University Medical Center) as a new graduate was very challenging. The step between school and real-life nursing was rather daunting. I figured that if this work environment was difficult, then working in the field would be even more demanding. I needed to get to a point where I felt comfortable in my role. Despite these initial feelings, I spoke with my manager about my plans. Later, I remember seeing my name on a Post-it® in his office stating "Naomi - Africa - 2 years." Thankfully he was very supportive of my plan, because his strong recommendation was a critical factor in being accepted into the pool of volunteers 2 years later.

I completed my first year as a new nurse—often feeling overwhelmed and looking like "a deer caught in headlights" according to a colleague. I decided to check in with MSF to see if I was on track to apply the following year. I learned about an MSF recruiting event planned to coincide with *A Refugee Camp in the Heart of the City* exhibit being held in Milwaukee. I flew up and excitedly visited the refugee camp exhibit. It was well designed and forced me to take a deeper look at access to care, specifically for those affected by war. I had spent a lot of time thinking about access to care with respect to poverty, but had not thought about displacement due to conflict. The idea of people running from burning villages to escape rape and murder with nothing but the clothes on their backs had never really been part of my thought process with respect to "helping" people. Even though I had read about refugee camps on the Internet, it didn't really click—until I saw the exhibit—that people in refugee camps need everything: shelter, basic and advanced health care, mental health care, disease prevention, nutrition assistance, and access to drinkable water. After visiting the exhibit, I felt emotionally drained and uneducated despite my best efforts to be informed. However, I remained dedicated to learning more about refugee populations and being part of humanitarian relief efforts.

I attended the MSF recruitment event and spoke with a representative about strategies to strengthen my application. She told me I needed to start working as charge nurse and to take on training responsibilities of new staff and nursing students. She also indicated that additional experience abroad and French language skills would increase my chances of getting an interview. She warned me that the process would be challenging. The grim but enlightening experience at the exhibit and the exchange with the recruiter made me even more determined to work for the organization. It also showed me that I still had a simplistic view of aid work and global access to health care. Little did I know, 1 year and 3 months later I would be working in a refugee camp as an MSF nurse.

As soon as I got back to the hospital, I had another meeting with my manager. After seeing the refugee camp exhibit and learning about the millions of displaced people in the world, I knew I needed to do the absolute maximum to be accepted for a mission. I asked if I could start taking on more training responsibilities, work as charge nurse, and also take a month off to go to Nepal for a volunteer opportunity. I was naturally nervous to take on the role of charge nurse, but I was determined to succeed in all the areas where I had to develop myself in order to go on a mission. After 8 months of successful work as a charge nurse, training new staff and students, studying French, reading everything I could about humanitarian aid work, and spending several weeks volunteering in a rural clinic outside of Chitwan, Nepal, I applied to MSF, with some hesitation. The hesitation came as a result of the experiences I had while working and traveling in Nepal. I questioned if I was mentally prepared for humanitarian aid work, because the living conditions for this volunteer opportunity were harsher than I had ever experienced. I lived in a small village with a charming

Nepalese family where there was very limited electricity, one pump with running water for 15 people, no transportation other than by foot or bike, limited English, two small meals per day consisting mainly of daal (spiced yellow lentils) and vegetables, very sick patients, a lot of female inequality, and limited resources in the small clinic where I had been assigned.

The culture shock was intense. For example, one night we did not have the usual 2 hours of electricity and Kopela, the mother of the family, and I were both on our period. As a result, we were not allowed in the kitchen, so we sat on the floor in the hallway peeling potatoes by candlelight so her sons could cook them for dinner. That moment was almost my breaking point, but I had to accept the cultural differences or I would come off as impolite in their home. To make matters more difficult, the clinic director where I volunteered was sexist and unprofessional with me and the other female staff members. His methods for treating patients were abstract. He had no interest in having a dialogue with me concerning differences in patient care between our two countries, despite several attempts on my part. We mostly assessed patients with the common cold, sinusitis-like conditions, tuberculosis, nonhealing wounds due to poor management—in my opinion—and leprosy. The work was interesting, but I did not really contribute to the betterment of the population. I did, however, learn how to choose my battles and embrace the experience for what it was.

I had never lived or worked in this type of environment and it was difficult, exhausting, and above all depressing. During the trip, I began to appreciate why MSF has such rigorous standards for their pool of volunteers. I questioned if I could handle extreme cultural differences and difficult living situations while meeting my professional responsibilities for more than the few weeks I had just experienced.

On my way back to Kathmandu, I contemplated my next steps. While stuck in traffic, I saw an MSF Land Rover with a seriously awesome and tough female MSF worker standing with several national staff team members. I thought to myself, "It's a sign; I should go ahead and apply!" I decided that one bizarre, albeit important, volunteer experience should not alter my goals. I submitted my application 1 month after my return from Nepal.

To my absolute delight, I was accepted into the pool of volunteers. Honestly, it felt like being drafted into the National Basketball Association (NBA), but for humanitarian aid workers! To be given the opportunity to work with the organization that I admire so much was an honor that I still feel today. The duration of the process was 7 months from submission of my application to departure for a mission. This is actually pretty quick considering I didn't speak much French and was a first-time mission nurse. The process involved answering a lot of questions via essay, two trips to New York for intense interviews and orientation meetings, and several months of waiting for an assignment. Being accepted by MSF was one of the most difficult professional hurdles I had passed until I got to the field.

THE LONG-AWAITED MISSION

I had worked for years toward what became an all-consuming goal to provide critically needed care to populations with vast medical needs in some of the most desperate situations. I was finally called to fill the post of nurse on a medical mission with the organization I had yearned to work for since my volunteer days in Tanzania. For the 2 years leading up to working with MSF, my focus had been on getting mentally and professionally prepared. All of the previous international volunteer experiences were important steps in my development as a future humanitarian aid worker. However, I gained a lot more from them in terms of understanding the complexities of the world around me than I actually gave to people who needed help. This was not the case during my first assignment, or the other missions that followed—where I learned in equal proportion to the aid I provided.

It had been almost 9 years since my curiosity in politics lit the long path toward international aid work in Africa. At long last, I found myself on the way to Uganda to work as the nurse manager of a cholera treatment center and an outpatient department in a refugee camp. Since that first mission, I have accepted three additional assignments: a meningitis vaccination program in Nigeria, a postwar hospital in Sri Lanka, and a measles vaccination program in the Democratic Republic of the Congo. All missions were less than 4 months in duration because they were classified as "emergency" interventions, meaning the teams work nonstop to manage the situation until it is stable or the time sensitive task (example: vaccination before the rainy season) is completed.

After being notified of the Uganda assignment, I had just 4 days to get my final affairs in order before heading to the New York office for a departure briefing. Fortunately MSF has an abundance of field protocols. I was given a cholera treatment protocol to read during the flight along with mission and country specific documents including context of the mission, security concerns, and a job description. MSF has a highly skilled team of personnel who manage arrangements for the expatriates before, during, and after an assignment. Before going on mission, I had not thought about the enormous level of coordination required between multiple groups of people in multiple countries:

human resources, logistics, security, communications, fundraisers, mission leaders, project leaders, local leaders, other NGO's, local staff, legal departments, medical specialists, financial coordinators, ministries of health, and the government of the country of mission. I was simply focused on doctors and nurses helping people in need, similar to what I had seen in my prior volunteer experiences. I hadn't considered how teams (often operating in war zones and catastrophes) get all their supplies or how they work in another country with respect to that country's laws. I was beyond naïve. Reality set in quickly. I managed to handle the tremendous work environment in which emergency humanitarian aid happens. I learned to appreciate the complexity of communication and team dynamics required to help people.

UGANDA AND A DIFFERENT UNDERSTANDING OF REALITY

The following (slightly edited) email to my family gives a quick sense of my initial feelings about the mission:

> The work here is *insane*! I flew from NYC into Kampala, and yes I saw the huge Lake Victoria, which is so beautiful. Then I had a 1-hour drive to the MSF house where I slept almost instantly and then had several meetings that evening for my trip the next morning. I left with an MSF-borrowed UNICEF ambulance in which I rode to Mbarara with medical supplies and a cold box with hepatitis B vaccinations for several women who had been raped before fleeing the Congo. After the 4-hour drive cramped in a two-and-a-half seat vehicle with two very pleasant Ugandan men, I met the first team member who had no clue I was coming. She also had no idea I was bringing a huge load of drugs and supplies. She was REALLY angry because of the lack of communication. To make room I had to help move all the boxes into a hotel supply room, which was difficult considering I was jet lagged, starving, and had just met these people. Then it was off to Kobingo, my living location for the mission. To my surprise, we drove right past it and went straight to work in Nakivali. Upon arrival I saw two large areas with semipermanent structures surrounded by protective walls, guards at each entry point, and several cows. One structure is the cholera treatment center; the other is the outpatient department. There is no electricity, no generator, and no running water. I went directly to a staff meeting and met everyone I would be working with and/or managing. I'm supervising nurse practitioners (4), registered nurses (6), nurse aids (6) who have the right to insert IVs and pass meds, cholera control sprayers (6) who go out into the refugee camp to spray contaminated areas in order to decrease cholera transmission, a

chlorinator (1) who makes all the solutions, cleaners (6), and for the first month all the watchmen on duty (16). I'm also in charge of the pharmacy, which involves managing the entire inventory including ordering drugs.

Our expatriate team is composed of six members: a project coordinator/ER doctor from the United States, a field doctor from Germany, one logistician (she hasn't said where she is from), a logistics administrator from Japan, a watsan (water/sanitation) from France, and me. We work from 7 a.m. until 6 p.m. every day and sometimes we work on Sunday if there is an emergency. The cholera seems to be under control and now that we are entering the dry season it may be done. The food is simple: beans and rice every day and sometimes goat meat or fish and *chipatis*. Power is available in the living quarters, which are located 40 minutes outside of the refugee settlement. There is no running water or normal toilet. Oh! I got out of working Christmas back home, but I made up for it by working Christmas here. Thankfully it was a laid back day!

I have to admit that I'm working harder than I've ever worked in my life. I finally became sick this week, which was inevitable considering the work load. Fortunately I got sent to Mbarara for a 24-hour rest period, hence my ability to send an e-mail. If the cholera stays under control and there are no major dysentery outbreaks (a problem last week), things should start to get a little better. On average, about 90 refugees come by bus from the border every other day. They are processed by UNHCR (United Nations High Commission for Refugees) and the Ugandan government. The UNHCR gives out plastic tenting material and non-food items, the World Food Program dispenses food items, and we provide medical care. When plots of land are organized the families are moved from the temporary settlement area near our clinic to Juru for a chance to set up a "home." Even though the cholera seems to have diminished, MSF is staying on while the government processes all the people coming from the border (Ishaha) camp and arranges for ongoing care.

What I didn't share in this e-mail was my level of responsibility or the connections formed with the expat/national staff colleagues and the refugees with whom I worked. When I started this mission I went from working in a U.S. hospital as an intermittent charge nurse/bedside nurse on a 32-bed step-down unit to a nurse manager of an outpatient department where at least 100 consultations were performed per day and a cholera treatment center that had several patients at any given time. I was responsible for staff management, scheduling, payroll (along with the logistic administrator), enforcing compliance with MSF protocols, training and teaching of the staff (often along with the expatriate doctor), and maintaining the pharmacy. I was also involved in patient advocacy and coordination of care with respect to getting assistance from other groups for special patient situations, such as coordinating a transfer to Mbarara for patients bitten by rabid dogs, finding living arrangements for orphaned children with posttraumatic stress disorder

> (PTSD), trying to relocate two women who had been held against their will in a man's refugee tent for several weeks before finally managing to escape, and I was responsible for getting baby formula and medications for a woman who had been raped and just tested positive for HIV. The list was endless.

The connections that I formed with national and expat staff were extremely interesting and dynamic. The MSF expat staff was filled with intelligent, hardworking, inspiring, confident, head strong, selfless people. We all came from diverse cultural backgrounds with different types of training and professional experience, but we were all focused on the same goal: providing the best possible care and assistance to arriving refugees. At times we did not always agree on a plan of action or have the same ideas about how to achieve our objectives, but with nightly discussions and great leadership from the project coordinator we stayed on the same page once decisions were made.

I learned a lot about effective communication and the importance of effective team dynamics from my interactions with the expat staff, but I learned even more from the national staff with respect to cultural sensitivity. We had excellent medical protocols in place based on the MSF field guidelines, but in the end, there were certain situations where knowing the local culture and medical practice (what was accepted and what was taboo) made the difference in how to proceed with treatment. I learned that Congolese and Ugandan nurses have very strong assessment skills, a flexible and creative nature when it comes to nursing with limited resources, a professional and inquisitive work manner, and a "can do" attitude even when they themselves have recently fled their homes to escape attacks from rebel groups. Without the expertise of local health professionals, we would not have been able to provide culturally appropriate care. MSF's commitment to hire and promote national staff to high level leadership positions within the organization makes it even more effective at providing the best possible care in the field.

Though the cholera outbreak was the primary reason for the presence of our team, we saw more patients coming to the outpatient department as the cholera cases decreased. We diagnosed and treated high numbers of malaria, upper respiratory infections, painful dental infections, diarrhea (noncholera), foot abscesses, eminent births, rapes with concern of sexually transmitted infections' and HIV, malnutrition, burns, PTSD, and ruptures in treatment of HIV and tuberculosis. Aside from these medical problems, the biggest necessity was potable water and mental health support. The only source of water was a large lake several hours away by foot. The water and sanitation team treated and transported water every other day to large bladders located at various sites throughout the refugee camp. However, as people were relocated to their plots of land, it became quite obvious that more had to be done to increase access to potable water. Access to clean water is essential not only because people need water to live, but also to diminish threats of disease outbreak (often cholera) due to poor hygiene. It was clear that access to water was becoming a project that extended beyond the scope of the acute cholera intervention.

The same can be said with respect to the need for psychological support for newly arrived refugees. The doctor and I worked with many women whose husbands had been murdered, they had been raped, their homes had been burned, and some of their children had been displaced or killed. They had severe PTSD, which in some cases seriously affected their ability to take care of their children, who were often quite sick. We were able to help one woman's children get desperately needed medical care and temporary placement with another woman who had been in the camp for years. We tried to help the mother but she needed more specific psychological resources than was available at the time. One of the MSF staff nurses took in several orphaned children. She had fled the Congo years ago after her husband was killed by rebels. She often spoke about the mental health needs of the children and asked if we could do something to address the issue. MSF has a strong program for psychological support in these situations. However, we did not have a psychologist on our team because we had only been approved to work in the country under the scope of cholera.

After 3 months of providing medical assistance to a transitioning population, the emergency phase of the mission came to an end. Another MSF section was approved (by the government) to provide longer-term assistance to the population with respect to access to water and psychological support. Our team held several mobile clinics for people who had relocated 5 to 7 miles away from the outpatient department. The project coordinator made an assessment of the ability of other NGOs to provide longer-term medical care in the area. We spent 2 days breaking down the cholera treatment center and the outpatient department. We said goodbye to our national staff colleagues during a big goodbye party. For me, the party and the goodbyes were bittersweet because I had grown close to the staff. I had eaten in some of their homes, I knew their children, and overall I had a glimpse of their harsh reality. It was hard to leave them knowing they were now out of a job with limited options for the near future. Many of them spoke of returning home once things were more peaceful in their villages or of seeking employment with the arriving MSF section.

REFLECTIONS

The information I have shared regarding my time in a refugee camp has touched on several themes, which could be greatly expanded. To delve into the nuances of each of my missions would require a few more pages and a lot more vulnerability on my part. However, what I would like to share is that I absolutely loved working in Uganda and that is why I continue to go on missions with MSF. Though the assignment at the refugee camp was challenging, I was mentally prepared for the work and the living conditions. My nursing process skills, my experience as a charge nurse, trainer of new staff, and mentor to students as well as my travels prior to going on mission prepared me well to manage whatever was thrown my way. While in Uganda, I learned a lot about how to be more effective in my role as an expat nurse supervisor. I adopted three golden rules, which have proven to be extremely helpful in all of my assignments:

- Listen more than you speak, because you may not know as much as you think you do and you need to understand the context or the culture; listening is a great way to learn.
- Be a team player, even when you feel like hell, because chances are someone on your team feels worse than you do and he or she needs your support.
- Above all be flexible. Chances are you will have to do something outside of your job description or comfort zone. Everyone is busy doing something outside of their job description in order to keep the mission going effectively, so you have to do your part.

These three little golden rules often made the difference between sinking and swimming when situations became overwhelming, such as when coping with your own gastrointestinal(GI) illness, working for 24 hours straight without sleep, or having just witnessed the death of a 5-year-old child due to starvation.

Finally, I want to touch on the fact that while I was professionally prepared for my role in the field, I was not prepared for the human suffering I witnessed. No one can ever really prepare for this aspect of humanitarian aid work. I've witnessed a lot of children, adults, and geriatric patients suffer unimaginable atrocities as a direct result of war. I've worked at the bedside of children and adults whose limbs were missing or who were paralyzed due to bomb blasts during the end of the war in Sri Lanka. I've seen people (mostly children and the elderly) die because of malaria, malnutrition, diarrhea, typhoid, and other preventable and or treatable diseases. I've stayed at the bedside with people as they cried upon learning that someone they love had been killed or could not be located. I held the hand of a crying woman because it was her birthday and she didn't feel she had the right to live because her mother had been killed by a bomb that had been dropped on their home. Sadly, there are millions of deeply tragic stories like these. Unfortunately, NGOs are sometimes denied access to conflict zones resulting in deaths, which could have been prevented if access to care had been granted sooner. To be in the presence of such intense suffering is humbling and difficult to cope with for any health care provider, but the need for assistance outweighs the difficulty individuals or organizations may face in order to provide care. On a personal level, I never knew how hard I could work, tirelessly, until I witnessed this type of suffering. It awakened a whole new level of "providing care" that I had not known before and it made me a better nurse both abroad and at home.

The key message I wish to convey is that people are suffering all around the world in unimaginable ways and they need help from nurses. People who are suffering need help from everyone, but since I am a nurse I can say for certain that they definitely need help from nurses! I say this because it is often the nurse who is at the bedside when a patient is suffering, more so than any other health care provider. Not only is alleviating suffering an important part of our job, but it goes hand in hand with our training in critical thinking, team work, good communication, and compassion. It is our action as a result of our training combined with our compassion that helps to decrease suffering.

COMING HOME

The most difficult aspect of humanitarian relief work, for me, is the time spent working in the United States between missions. After spending months working in a management role with huge responsibility outside the normal scope of bedside nursing with people who were suffering in ways I had never seen, the adjustment was surreal. During my first week back at work I remember seeing all the crisp clean bed linen being changed when it wasn't dirty, the tubes coming out of every orifice of my patients' bodies to go along with several different IV infusions with top-of-the-line medications, and a lot of impatience from patients and family members. This was a stark contrast to putting in IVs while using my headlamp and counting drips to get the infusion correct for a patient lying on a piece of plastic sheeting on the ground who had walked at least 5 miles for treatment and had been found collapsed on the side of the dirt road.

I kept thinking to myself that most of the people I cared for in the United States would have already died if they lived in the countries where I went on medical mission. In those locations, people died from very treatable and preventable diseases such as malnutrition and malaria, not advanced vascular diseases or cancer or lack of access to timely transplants. This is exactly the opposite thought I had while working on mission. I often thought, "It doesn't have to be this way, these children would probably be healthy had they been born in a different location on the planet." Trying to reconcile the inequities in access to care based on where one is born is not possible; hence the reason I continue to go on mission. Everyone deserves access to affordable care regardless of birthplace, race, ethnicity, religion, political situation, or the amount of money in their pocket. In some places there is simply *no access* to care. It doesn't matter how much money someone has if they live in an area with an inadequate or nonexistent health care infrastructure due to government corruption, poverty, or war.

That said, the amount of money in one's pocket does directly affect access to care in the United States. Although systems to assure access to care exist, without sufficient means, proper insurance coverage, preventative care, or government assistance many patients fall through the cracks. They do not seek care until their pathology is advanced and, as a result, they require significant and costly interventions. It's this group of people who are the most vulnerable to suffering.

Barriers to access to care, whether one lives in a war-torn country with severely limited resources or in the United States where the complexities of the health care infrastructure often block access, are unacceptable. Human suffering is human suffering. The context may be different for each patient. We may perceive that the level of suffering felt by one person is less severe than it is for someone else. However, none of this matters to the person who is suffering—it is a nightmare within the context of his or her life, culture, and reality. I had to learn to accept that the patients I care for in the United States live in a completely different world than those in other countries where I have worked. I had to learn how to be sensitive to this difference despite seeing what I consider to be the most horrible suffering I've ever witnessed while working in the field with MSF.

It is hard to compare the two different realities. I had to accept that I can't judge another person's suffering. But, I can use my nursing skills to provide the most competent, compassionate, and culturally sensitive care possible to help return—to some state of normalcy—a life turned upside down—regardless of the patient's location on this planet.

My journey started more than a decade ago and I find that I still have more questions than answers. What I know is that anyone with the desire to help vulnerable populations can start in his or her own community. Just look around and you will quickly see people who need your help. When you have done your homework, venture outside of your comfort zone and reach out to the global community. There aren't enough nurses out there to meet critical nursing needs. Once you witness suffering, you will be forever changed. This change will push you to be the best nurse you can be in order to serve those who need your help, regardless of the sacrifices you must make to help them.

4

A Nurse's Conflict

Care Diverted During a Coup

ANNA FREEMAN

Editor's Note: I have known Anna Freeman since she was a young girl playing with my children. It has been a pleasure to watch her mature into a capable and compassionate woman. Her report of working as a field nurse with Médecins Sans Frontières (MSF) during a time of violent conflict raises a number of ethical issues—ones that nurses have grappled with for generations. We hear so much about MSF in the news but little about the personal experiences of its workers. I am honored that within the MSF organization there is support for the desire of both Naomi (Chapter 3) and Anna to share their stories with us.

Pediatrics and Pediatric Intensive Care are where my nursing career started over 10 years ago. Both were fulfilling and I enjoyed working with critically ill children very much. After a few years of hospital nursing in the United States, I began working in international medical humanitarian aid, with an organization called Médecins Sans Frontières/Doctors Without Borders (MSF). I have worked with MSF for several years, in several different countries. At different times and in different places, these experiences have been interesting, challenging, and rewarding. Here, I describe my experience working with MSF in the Central African Republic (CAR) in the spring of 2013, during a tumultuous period when its government was overthrown in a coup d'état. In this chapter, all names have been changed.

AN UNPLANNED BEGINNING

I am sitting in the front passenger seat of one of MSF's trademark white land cruisers as we bump along a broken road. I am wearing a white MSF vest that is five sizes too big but has ample pockets for my notebook, staff roster, MSF medical guidelines, pens, sunscreen, security documents, a copy of my passport, telephone numbers of team members, and my MSF identity card. The driver next to me is a Central African named Didier. Behind us, on the long benches in the back of the car, is the mobile clinic medical staff: two midwives, two nurses, and a pharmacy technician—all Central Africans. Two hundred yards ahead of us is another MSF land cruiser, this one carrying a driver and Giovanni, an Italian logistician. Their car is packed full of medications and equipment—everything from simple oral malaria treatment to intravenous drugs that halt preterm labor to plastic tables, chairs, and garbage bins—that we will need to perform a full day's clinic. Today, we expect a typical clinic, with over 100 pediatric consultations and 50 prenatal visits.

We are heading south from the town of Sibut, where we are based and where other members of our team are working in an abandoned government hospital. Sibut is in the middle of CAR, about 100 miles north of Bangui, the capital. We cross a bridge that takes us over a small river. It is the dry season and the river is low, but we can see women washing their clothes and bathing their children in the brown water. About a mile past the bridge, we pass through a police checkpoint, now manned by members of a rebel group that has been slowly gaining control of more and more territory in CAR. The Seleka, as they are called, have recently taken over the towns along this road, and with them, the road itself. It is one of very few paved roads in the country and is an important thoroughfare because it provides access from Bangui to Chad, CAR's neighbor to the north. Several rebels dressed in camouflage and bearing automatic rifles and handguns man this checkpoint. They wave us through and greet the drivers in Arabic and Sango, the national language of CAR, as we slowly drive under the barrier that they lift for us. Moments later, our car's high-frequency radio comes to life. Idris, our Sierra Leonean project coordinator, is calling from our hospital base, yelling to be heard over the static. He tells us to turn back immediately, explaining that the mobile clinic has been cancelled due to insecurity in our immediate area. I call the other car's radio to make sure they've heard the conversation, and Didier makes a careful three-point turn to head back north to Sibut.

I turn to my team, who sit silently listening to the exchange between Idris and me. We discuss what we'll do instead of running the mobile clinic; the midwives will lend a hand in the hospital, one helping with gynecological and prenatal examinations and the other assisting the traditional birth attendants with deliveries. The nurses will assist in the inpatient and outpatient pediatrics departments. The pharmacy tech will work on organizing our stock and help out in the hospital pharmacy, if need be. I plan to work on the statistics for the week. I arrived only a few days ago and need to familiarize myself with the caseload for each practitioner and with the diseases that we are seeing. We all assume that we will carry on with the mobile clinic the following day; in the meantime, this is a welcome opportunity to get organized. At this point, we do not realize that over the weekend the Seleka will successfully take down the government.

BACKGROUND

This is my second assignment in the CAR. I have already worked as a nurse with MSF for several years, with assignments in the Democratic Republic of the Congo (DRC), Haiti, and South Sudan. I've provided care for people who have been displaced due to conflict, victims of war trauma, women with high-risk pregnancies, malnourished and critically ill children, and people with HIV and tuberculosis, and responded to outbreaks of preventable illnesses such as measles and cholera. I have been working in western CAR for the past 5 months, on a different MSF project, and only recently arrived in Sibut.

The CAR, as the name suggests, is located in the middle of the African continent. It is a former French colony, and although it gained independence in 1960, a heavy-handed French presence afterward prevented the country from developing along with its neighbors. President François Bozize came to power during a coup in 2003. The country has been relatively calm during the past few years, but various militias have recently been stirring. Several small militias in the northeastern part of the country have banded together, forming a coalition that they call the Seleka, meaning "alliance" in Sango. In official communications with CAR's media, Seleka made clear their objective to overthrow Bozize, who they saw as a corrupt leader who unfairly favored the citizens of CAR that are from his region and tribe. By late 2012, the Seleka had begun to slowly move across the country toward Bangui, ending in the coup the week I arrived in Sibut.

MSF has been working in CAR for many years, with multiple projects throughout the country. Our mandate is to provide medical assistance to populations living in distress, which includes people living in danger of armed conflict, epidemic diseases, health care exclusion, or natural disasters. In CAR, as in many other countries that have a history of conflict and a poorly developed health system, MSF maintains several projects, which may be open for months or years, and also stands ready to respond to emergencies as they arise.

As the Seleka advanced upon Bangui in December 2012, MSF monitored the humanitarian situation along their path. When the rebels settled in Sibut, MSF sent a team to assess the health consequences of the rebel presence. This team found three major causes for concern. First, the rebel presence forced most of the qualified health care professionals at Sibut Hospital and in the area health centers to flee to Bangui or into the bush. No doctors or midwives remained in the region. The hospital and health centers were being run entirely by a handful of registered nurses, assisted by nursing assistants and traditional birth attendants with no formal education. Second, all of the health facilities had been completely looted during the attacks, and some of the buildings damaged during fighting. Most had no drugs or supplies to test and treat patients. Additionally, as the road from Bangui (where all medications and equipment for the hospitals and health centers in CAR originate) was taken over by the rebels, there was no possibility for delivery of new drugs or equipment. Third, most of the population had fled and did not feel safe traveling. In short: people were unable to seek care due to insecurity. If they did make it to a health facility, there were few or no qualified health care professionals and no drugs with which to treat them. This is a typical scenario when political instability is coupled with violence.

THE SIBUT PROJECT

In light of these findings, MSF opened the Sibut project, with a focus on providing care for young children and women of child-bearing age. These two populations are the most vulnerable to illness and have higher rates of morbidity and mortality than older children and men. The project had two main goals: to provide high-quality primary care to women and children in Sibut and in the surrounding area, and to provide high-quality secondary health care at Sibut Hospital for those patients needing inpatient services. In order to achieve these goals, we would provide support to Sibut Hospital and run a mobile clinic to support the six health centers north and south of Sibut. At the hospital, MSF added temporary qualified staff from Bangui, brought in drugs and equipment, implemented easy-to-follow protocols, and maintained a continuous medical presence in order to address complicated or life-threatening illnesses or injuries. As our target population was women and young children, we focused our support in the outpatient pediatric clinic, women's health clinic, inpatient pediatrics, maternity, and operating theater. Given the context, we were also ready to respond to surgical emergencies related to violence. Sigrid, a German physician, was responsible for the hospital-based activities.

MSF also opened a mobile clinic to serve people living along the road that connects Bangui to the Chadian border via Sibut. The aim of this team of nurses and midwives was to serve women and young children who were living or seeking refuge along this thoroughfare. The mobile clinic nurses and midwives planned to visit six clinics per week and work with any remaining staff (or volunteers from the community) to provide pediatric and antenatal consultations. Children needing to be hospitalized or women with indications of complicated pregnancies were referred to the Sibut Hospital and transported with us at the end of each day. I was in charge of this component of our project.

This project is typical of the work MSF does throughout the world. Readily available and experienced field volunteers are able to dispatch quickly to countries and regions with changing political and humanitarian contexts, evaluate the health needs within those areas, and build projects that address those needs. A well-organized and reactive logistical department makes this possible via emergency kits to treat victims of new violence, outbreaks of epidemic disease, or displaced persons on extremely short notice. Standardized and evidence-based medical protocols and pharmacy supply lists facilitate MSF's reactivity and ability to provide high-quality care, even in tenuous situations like this one in CAR.

CONFLICT ERUPTS

The next three days are chaotic and tense. I feel as if they are flying by and yet I am also acutely aware of each minute that passes. On Friday, we are awakened at daybreak to more rebels leaving for Bangui. They pile onto pick-up trucks and fire their guns into the air as they drive away from Sibut. The rebels have bases on either side of the hospital, so their leave taking is extremely loud and seems to come from all directions. Many of the national staff are from Bangui and are worried about their families. They use our satellite phone to call home. We hear from them that Bangui is tense, with government forces preparing to fight. One midwife has a brother in the Presidential Guard. She cannot reach him, and her family hasn't heard from him, either. They are worried that members of the Guard have fled, in fear of attacks on Bozize in the coming days. If her brother has fled, she will likely never see him again, as he will be forced to live in exile; if not, he faces almost certain death due to his loyalty to Bozize.

Over breakfast, we listen to Radio France International (RFI), hoping for more information on rebel movements, and we hear that there is major fighting just south of Sibut. Later in the day, RFI reports that the Seleka has taken two more towns in between Sibut and Bangui. Our head of mission calls to inform us that the Seleka has also attacked an MSF hospital north of Sibut, stealing drugs, equipment, money, and holding the expats at gunpoint.

We were scheduled to visit a clinic south of Sibut that day but our plans are canceled because of proximity to the front lines. Instead, the mobile clinic team and I prepare for an influx of patients, expecting the Seleka to send their soldiers to us if they are injured. We prepare a mass casualty kit: a large metal trunk with the medicines and equipment to treat approximately 50 war-wounded soldiers. We prep the small operating theater with resuscitation materials and equipment for laparotomy. While our project's intended beneficiaries are civilians, we would never deny medical care to wounded soldiers. MSF offers assistance to people based on need, irrespective of race, religion, gender, or political affiliation. We also remain neutral, not taking sides during a conflict. If the fighting continues, we anticipate that the rebels will, indeed, require our assistance.

In the afternoon, we receive two soldiers from a neighboring country with gunshot wounds to the thigh, brought to us in Seleka trucks. They tell us they were shot by government forces, approximately 20 miles south of Sibut. We had heard that troops from neighboring countries were supporting the government, so this news is surprising. Their wounds are too extensive for us to fully treat; they need emergency surgery to fix their badly broken femurs. We do not have a surgeon, only a nurse who has been trained to do cesarean sections and simple abdominal repairs. There is no possibility for transfer to a hospital in Bangui, as doing so would require crossing the front lines. We manually reduce their fractures and monitor them closely for bleeding. We also treat their pain, dress their wounds to prevent infection, and create makeshift casts out of cardboard and gauze. This is the best we can do with limited resources.

We take time to hide our valuables in case we, too, are robbed. Sigrid and I find spots for our iPods and cameras, and tuck our cash beneath our mattresses. Our cooks make a special trip around town, to stock up on whatever food items they can find, in case we are unable to leave the base in the coming days.

When we awake on Saturday, Sibut is eerily quiet. Staff and patients are on edge as we wait for news from Bangui. We listen to RFI and learn that there has been more fighting along the road in between Sibut and Bangui, and that a South African helicopter has been shot down by rebel forces. We receive a phone call from our head of mission telling us that the rebels are still advancing on the capital. Tension grows among our national staff as we start working.

Before heading to the wards, I quickly send my family an e-mail. It happens to be my father's birthday and he is retiring after a 30-year career as an epidemiologist. A party is planned for that evening with my childhood friends and family gathering together. It's surreal to be thinking of them celebrating as we scramble to treat rebel soldiers with a dwindling supply of drugs and equipment. I both wish that I were with them and am glad to be with my team in CAR.

Partway through the morning, we hear loud trucks and gunfire as a convoy of Seleka barrels into the hospital. A code red is called—all hands on deck for a mass casualty. Within minutes, the admissions area is overflowing with rebels. There are dozens of people; they have taken every bed. Others are on the floor in between each bed, on the walkway outside the rooms, and still others wait outside on makeshift stretchers (raw planks of wood). Uninjured rebel soldiers are running around and yelling for help for their friends. It is chaos.

Quickly, we divvy up tasks to manage the injured. The medical staff divides into teams with Sigrid or Christophe, a Central African physician, passing by each patient to evaluate their wounds and plan treatment. The nurses and midwives take different rooms and do quick assessments to identify the most critically wounded, and then start tending to injuries. The members of the logistics staff work on crowd control, circulating through each room to ask noninjured people to wait outside while we treat the patients. They also ensure that the soldiers respect rules about guns. The soldiers are heavily armed with automatic rifles and often handguns. Noninjured soldiers waited at the gate of the hospital holding an armful of weapons that belong to the soldiers being treated.

Many of the injured soldiers are stoic. They respond to questions when they can in French or through interpreters in Arabic or Sango. It is surprising to approach a man who is waiting calmly on a mat in between beds, then to find that he has been shot multiple times, with in-and-out wounds to his shoulders, arms, and legs. As we triage and treat people, and as crowd control becomes more effective, the rooms with patients actually become rather quiet as we work our way around.

One of the injured men is a Seleka general that had been stationed in Sibut and with whom we had been in close communication prior to their advance on Bangui. He has been shot in the thigh and his femur is badly broken. We gave him pain medicine and antibiotics and try to set his leg as best we can with our very limited supplies. In his pain-medicine-induced delirium, he babbles about their strategy to descend on Bangui and talks about needing to get back to the front lines to support his troops. Although we are caring for many different Seleka members, it's unnerving to provide care for the general.

Our security system includes daily contact with all of the village leaders in Sibut, including the Catholic priests, the imams at the Muslim mosque, the village elders, and the militia leaders. The mayor of Sibut fled when the Seleka took over, otherwise, we would have been in contact with him, too. We all knew the general and relied on him to communicate to us when the security situation in the area changed. Further, we depended on him to control his troops when they got riled up or when they started drinking. It was therefore unsettling to see such a powerful man laid up in a hospital bed, and especially in his drug-induced delirium.

As I care for him, he learns my name, and then refers to all of the female nurses as Madame Anna. The other soldiers in the room whisper to us that he had actually been shot in the abdomen several times, causing his intestines to fall out. They say he used magic to quickly put his intestines back into his stomach and to move his injury to his leg, which they see as being a much less dangerous spot for a gunshot wound. This sort of magical thinking is common. Many of the soldiers wear amulets with bits of the Koran inside for protection, and some have small vials of water that has been charmed with protective powers against bullets.

The hospital is quiet but tense as we wait for news from Bangui and set up night shifts to tend to the new patients. Young women who are associated with the Seleka arrive with plates of food for the rebels—manioc paste and goat meat. The women hover over the injured men, fanning them and tending to them. They don't speak to us or acknowledge the medical team at all.

After daybreak on Sunday, we receive another convoy of injured Seleka. Our logistics team erects a canvas tent that we use to triage and treat these soldiers. Staff who worked overnight try to get some rest before joining us to continue treating the wounded. As we work in the tent, an uninjured soldier runs in, waving his rifle over his head and shouting in Arabic. Abdul, our driver who is attempting to control the crowd, interprets for us as the soldier makes his announcement.

He tells us that Bozize has fled and that the Seleka have taken over the government. The soldiers in the tent erupt in cheers. The Seleka in town start firing their guns into the air in celebration. It is loud and even closer than the gunfire we heard as the soldiers left for Bangui a few days ago. Sigrid and I hover near our mass casualty trunk. After several minutes, the shouting we hear turns from celebratory to angry. It's a frightening turn of events. Sigrid and I continue treating patients, staying low out of fear. We ask what the angry-sounding soldiers outside are saying, but it's difficult for anyone to hear them. The men we are treating speak limited French and cannot interpret for us. Finally, as the yelling grows louder, Sigrid and I leave the tent and run to our safe room, a small, enclosed room in our laboratory home that is packed with sandbags. As we take off at a run for the room, we hear the soldiers laughing at us. We are told later that they were mocking us for being scared of what were clearly nonthreatening gunshots and yelling.

That afternoon, the gunfire has calmed down, and we make rounds on the patients who had arrived over the previous 2 days. They are all in good spirits after hearing news of the successful coup d'état, and many of them ask Sigrid and me, through interpreters, if we are married, proposing on the spot. The men are clearly excited and joke with us and each other as we move from bed to bed. One of them has a bottle of cologne (in a bottle shaped like a grenade, which startles us as we approach his bed to assess him), which the men pass around to spritz on themselves.

A crowd suddenly appears in the ward, led by soldiers bearing rifles and yelling at the women who are tending to the male soldiers to leave the room. A well-dressed man asks us to gather around him for an announcement as Michel Djotodia, the head of the Seleka and self-proclaimed president of CAR, comes into the room. He is dressed in formal attire and is surrounded by bodyguards; a hush falls over the room as he enters and prepares to give a short speech. He begins by announcing that the Seleka have taken over the government of

CAR and that he is now the leader of the country. The soldiers cheer as he says this, while we listen in silence. He continues, talking about how different the country will be under his leadership, saying that the corruption that has shaped the Bozize presidency is over. He thanks MSF, telling us that without our care for his soldiers the Seleka would not have succeeded in taking Bangui. As he speaks, one of his assistants, who is holding a rocket launcher and has a satellite phone clipped to his pocket, records him on an iPad.

None of us is sure how to respond. We shake his hand, and those of his assistants, uneasily thanking him for the visit and nodding as he repeats how grateful he is to MSF for caring for his men. While we would never deny care to anyone, I am uncomfortable hearing his praise, as if our objective is to facilitate the work of a rebel group whose actions have injured and killed many, and whose actions will lead the country into an ongoing conflict.

As we continue to dress wounds and distribute medication to the soldiers at the hospital, I think of the women and children who are not receiving care in the mobile clinic, and those who cannot come to the hospital as they are too scared to leave their homes. We are unable to serve them due to the insecurity caused by the rebels who are now under our care. However, I realize that many of the soldiers come from circumstances just like the women and children we would normally be treating: extreme poverty, with few options for employment or upward mobility. Some have also been coerced into joining the rebel group. The medical needs of men in front of me are as important as those of the women and children in the area, but I regret that we cannot care for both at this time.

A NEW NORMAL

In the days after the coup, fighting continues in Bangui and along the road leading up to Sibut. We stay in the hospital, treating new civilian victims of violence and more injured rebel soldiers, while maintaining our hospital-based activities for women and children who are able to come in for treatment. The rebels living in Sibut revel in their victory, and we hear celebratory gunfire constantly. Another friendly general, a colleague of the man with the broken femur that we treated, comes and goes from Bangui. Whenever he is in town he meets with Idris or Ben, our new project coordinator who is British. They discuss the security situation in surrounding areas, and whether or not the rebels intend to stay in Sibut as they take more and more power in Bangui.

The jubilant atmosphere in Sibut is unsettling. As the rebels who live next to the hospital wave to us as in a neighborly way, we hear stories from our head of mission, on RFI, and from the families of our national staff in Bangui about Seleka's behavior in the capital. There is more and more fighting on the streets and people do not feel safe leaving their homes. The new president seems to have little control over his troops. In some neighborhoods, even staying home becomes unsafe as rebels rob civilians and institute a "disarmament program," an excuse to steal weapons from civilians for their own use. Additionally, members of the Seleka have started to fight among themselves, battling on the streets of Bangui over promotions, room and board, and other unknown disagreements.

The MSF office and two expat homes in Bangui are robbed. The office was empty when broken into, but it was thoroughly destroyed and all of the computers and other valuables taken. Houses are robbed more than once, with guns held to the heads of expats and national staff guards. Cars are stolen—the safe containing the project's cash and expat passports is taken. Other NGOs are also robbed, and almost all evacuate their entire expat teams. In towns all over CAR, project sites are robbed and expats and national staff are threatened. In Sibut, we are spared this, most likely because we continue to provide health care for injured rebels. One day, a hospital guard runs into our office to report that he has just seen two stolen MSF cars drive by, heading north and full of Seleka.

It is dispiriting to hear these stories and know that many of our colleagues are living in fear and being traumatized by the soldiers we are treating. While MSF works in many insecure environments, this level of looting, robbery, and threatened personnel is rare. The immense needs of the population motivate us to maintain our program and the others as much as possible, but the level of insecurity surpasses a typical MSF mission.

We watch as the rebels in our area turn over, and more and more soldiers are recruited. Many of the recruits are young, in their mid- to late-teens, and some are women. I never ask anyone about the women soldiers, but we speculate about the life of a female among the Seleka. The women are expected to train with the men and are issued automatic weapons, but they also work in the kitchen, preparing food for everyone, making tea, and often fanning the generals as they sit in the hot sun. The dynamic is disconcerting and likely unsafe, in many ways, for the women soldiers.

During the weeks after the coup, our mobile clinic remains on standby; the road going north and south of Bangui is too unsafe to travel regularly, especially with the current tendency of the Seleka to rob NGOs. While the risk of travel is apparent, I start to feel antsy at the hospital. Our mandate is to treat everyone, regardless of political affiliation, and I firmly believe that everyone has the right to quality health care, including members of rebel groups. Nevertheless, it is frustrating to be unable to reach the women and children that we were treating via the mobile clinic. Meanwhile, the soldiers are able to receive care as needed. Patients start to come to the hospital from farther and farther away (some walking over 10 miles to reach us), a dangerous undertaking that women and mothers can only justify when they or their children are already gravely ill. It is heartbreaking to receive dying babies and children with illnesses that would have been easily treated with earlier intervention.

TAKING CARE OF OURSELVES

During this calmer but still tense period in Sibut, we usually finish work between 6 and 7 p.m., often because the small room we use as an office is too uncomfortable to stay in for long. There is almost no circulation, as the windows to all of the rooms have sandbags in front of them in case of gunfire, and the hallways are filled with boxes of medications and cooking supplies for the expat kitchen. At night, the room fills with insects, which are attracted to the overhead light bulb and our computer screens. They form clouds that circulate in front of us, or hit the light bulb and die, falling onto our heads or down the backs of our shirts. The building is also full of rats, which scurry around at night and run over our feet while we try to work. Concentrating on our statistics or writing reports becomes difficult, so we move outside to have team meetings, listen to RFI, and try to relax.

We entertain ourselves by coming up with creative ways to cook with our very limited ingredients. The road from Bangui remains too dangerous to transport food, so we are eating up the remaining items in our small food stock and relying on what can be bought locally. Each MSF project is required to have an emergency food ration at all times, in case the expat team is required to bunker down in the safe room for an extended period. This trunk of store-bought canned foods tempts us every day as we eat what we have left, but we do not open it, knowing that we could find ourselves in worse circumstances at any point.

We can buy small antelopes to eat, which have been killed and then cooked whole over a fire, skin and hair intact. This is usually our only meat source (although as a vegetarian, I usually pass on this one). Occasionally, we can buy a live chicken or two, which our cooks or drivers kill. Chicken is incredibly expensive, though, and as the money in our cash box dwindles, it becomes more and more rare. However, we can often find eggs, and we are in the middle of avocado and mango season. We also have what seems to be a never-ending supply of manioc products: flour and leaves, which are staples in this part of the world. Luckily, we have a large bucket of rice that was brought to us from Bangui prior to the coup, along with a huge drum of palm oil. Day after day, our cooks prepare the same lunch: rice with the cooked antelope, scrambled eggs (with onions if we can get them), sliced avocados, a paste made from manioc flour called *boule*, and cooked manioc leaves. They spend the afternoon cleaning up the kitchen and doing the laundry since there isn't anything else to cook anyway. Our evening meal consists of leftovers from lunch—hence, the need to get creative.

Luckily, we have a few remaining items from Bangui: bread stored in a nonfunctioning refrigerator to keep it safe from rats, tomato sauce, pesto, popcorn kernels, mustard, soy sauce, and some limes. Sigrid masters making popcorn over a fire, and it becomes a favorite snack for a few days. We also make creative sandwiches combining the manioc, onions, antelope meat, and various Bangui condiments. One night, Sigrid and I grill a few slices of bread and make bruschetta with the jar of pesto. We eat it at a plastic table under the bright stars and enjoy talking about our lives at home and sharing stories from past missions. She and I work together every day, sharing a bedroom and a sense of isolation. We quickly become very close. Amazingly, we do not tire of each other during the 2 months spent side-by-side in CAR. After dinner, we quiz each other with our "portable Google": the pages at the front of a Moleskine calendar that have lists of measurement conversions, time zones, and different clothing sizes in the United States, Europe, and Great Britain. This provides more entertainment than one might expect, until we realize we've actually memorized the number of time zones between Greenwich Mean Time (GMT) and capital cities throughout the world. Sometimes we set up our portable cinema—a plastic table with someone's laptop and external hard drive—for movie night (the popcorn comes in handy on these nights). Since we do have power in the evening thanks to our generators, the best place for the portable cinema is either next to the poorly lit latrines or in the middle of the yard behind our building. On nights when gunfire is heavy, we abandon our movies and huddle in the doorway of the building until the shots die down.

BACK TO WORK

Our night at the movies is sometimes interrupted by the arrival of mass casualties, or by sick children in the pediatric ward. Sigrid and I alternate taking call, along with one national staff doctor and one nurse. When a child arrives at night and is gravely ill, or an already hospitalized child deteriorates, the pediatric nurse comes to get us at the gate to our building. Most of the hospital isn't lit since the hospital generators were stolen by the Seleka. Our generators provide light to the pediatric building and operating theater, when needed. This lack of light and the unpredictability of the soldiers living around the hospital require that one of our guards escorts us to pediatrics, holding a flashlight. We wear headlamps, which are useful if we need to start IVs or assess a patient.

When we receive mass casualties, it is almost always groups of Seleka who have crashed their trucks into each other or driven off the road. We continue to treat the injured Seleka in our triage tent, suturing their lacerations and setting broken bones, before they speed off again. We recognize the poorly disguised logos from the United Nations or other aid organization vehicles. One night, while we treat a group of about ten soldiers, our midwife leaves to tend to a woman who is having prolonged labor. She gives me a quick update on the soldier she is treating and asks me to continue dressing his wounds. As she walks away, the soldier becomes belligerent, yelling at her to come back immediately and accusing her of abandoning him. Through interpreters, we attempt to calm him down, quickly tending to his wounds but feeling nervous that his anger will escalate to violence. Luckily, he settles down and then turns on the charm, offering me yet another marriage proposal.

One night when I am on call, an 8-month-old baby is brought to the hospital with malaria and severe anemia. His hematocrit is measured using a rudimentary device that holds a small tube of blood you manually spin until the red blood cells separate from the rest of the blood. The hematocrit is read by comparing the tube to a small chart. In order for this to be done, a different guard from the hospital must go to the home of the laboratory technician, which fortunately is behind the hospital. Doing so, however, means that the guard must walk alone in the middle of the night past the rebel base, a courageous act in these circumstances. This night, the baby's hematocrit comes back at a dangerously low value. However, we cannot bank blood since we have no way of refrigerating the blood bags, and any patient needing a transfusion must receive a direct donation from a family member. This, of course, means that they must have a family member with them who has a compatible blood type and who is not infected with HIV, Hepatitis B or C, or syphilis. This is not always possible. The baby is not showing any signs of distress from his anemia, so I decide to observe him overnight and test his mother's blood if he starts to deteriorate.

Later, the nurse from pediatrics returns to the base and tells me that the mother of another patient is now ill. This time, the mother of a malnourished 2-month-old, with a complicated medical history of her own, is in shock. The young woman, the second wife of her husband, is HIV positive (as are her husband and his first wife). Unlike the first wife, she is not on treatment for her HIV, and when I arrive in pediatrics, she is hypothermic, unconscious, and having difficulty breathing. She is already receiving IV antibiotics for pneumonia, but I place another IV and give her IV glucose and a bolus of IV fluids. We wrap her in a survival blanket to attempt to warm her up, but she is having almost continuous diarrhea. Her husband and his first wife, who attentively care for her, prefer to keep her lightly covered in order to keep her clean. She regains partial consciousness, and panics, trying to pull out her IVs and pick up her baby, who is also attached to an IV and therefore difficult for her to manage. We give her an anxiolytic and place her baby in her arms, with her husband's first wife propping the two of them up. We attempt to give them privacy as a family, despite the shared room with other patients. Half an hour later, the husband reports that she has stopped breathing.

Over the years, as a nurse in the United States and abroad, I have seen many children and adults pass away. However, this woman's death is particularly sad for me. She was quite young, in her early 20s, and her death was entirely preventable. She died of an illness that could have been avoided, or with treatment could have been controlled for many years. I do not know if her baby was infected with HIV. She had delivered in the bush where they do not have access to even simple preventive therapies. This woman's illness and death were not a direct result of the Seleka or the fighting during the coup, but are emblematic of the nonfunctional health care system that exists in CAR. Her death is an indirect consequence of the fighting, which prevented her from seeking care in a timely manner.

Being with her family around the time of her death was a powerful experience; one that hasn't yet left me. I still acutely feel the frustration of being able to do so little for her, and the sorrow of her early departure, leaving such a tiny baby behind. But I hold on to the other memories from that night: her husband and his first wife tending to her lovingly as she fell ill and helping her to spend precious moments with her baby as she died. After her death, they buried her next to the hospital and continued caring for her baby, the first wife nursing him along with her own.

UNCERTAINTY CONTINUES

As the country becomes increasingly more unstable, we get word of Seleka destroying towns in the northwest of the country, particularly in the region where Bozize, the now exiled president, was raised. More and more rebels move south to Bangui and Sibut becomes calmer. As the road becomes less dangerous we see commerce trucks making the journey from Bangui to Chad and back. For the next couple of weeks, I join a team traveling to the northwest of the country to assess the situation since the coup. The news is disturbing, and MSF begins to develop intervention plans. But my time in CAR is coming to an end.

Sigrid, Ben, and I leave Sibut and spend 2 days in Bangui, writing project closure reports and compiling the data and pharmacy consumption figures from our activities. Bangui continues to deteriorate, as infighting among the Seleka increases and civilians defend their homes against marauding rebels. At night, gunshots echo around our house, but mostly they are far enough away that we do not feel scared.

I finally head home for a much-needed vacation. I stay in touch with Sigrid, Ben, and Giovanni. Ben stays in CAR for several more months, managing a new project in the northwestern part of the country. After taking holidays in Europe and the United States, Sigrid, Giovanni, and I all sign up for another mission with MSF. Giovanni is sent to the DRC to manage a vaccination campaign, and Sigrid returns to CAR to coordinate the medical activities for MSF country wide. I take a post in Haiti, managing a cholera response, and when that project closes, I head to Uganda to work in a refugee camp for Congolese refugees. Thanks to e-mail, we manage to stay in touch, and we send each other notes to describe our new projects, new living conditions, and new teams. Looking back over the time we spent together, it surprises me that it was only a few weeks. The bond that we share seems stronger than one that would normally come from such a short time together.

Working in CAR during this tumultuous period was the most challenging assignment I've ever had as I witnessed the horrific effects of conflict on the health of a population. Leaving Sibut, knowing that the needs there were still enormous, was extremely difficult. Working as a nurse in a conflict zone is both gratifying and frustrating. The needs are often much greater than what one individual can address, or what one organization can address, even one as well run and well funded as MSF. Learning to accept these limitations is something I continue to work on as I respond to new assignments and provide care for people living in distress.

5

Here Among Us

Caring for Migrant and Immigrant Patients in Rural United States

CANDACE KUGEL

Editor's Note: Candace Kugel reflects on her work as a family nurse practitioner and certified nurse-midwife with migrant farmworkers in a rural community in the United States. She demonstrates her passion to serve farmworkers through advocacy on a national scale in which she supports colleagues working in similar settings. She also describes short-term experiences in Latin America, echoing themes in Part II about weaving avocational endeavors into our work life.

GLOBAL HEALTH IN THE UNITED STATES

"Global health in the United States" is one of the simplistic descriptions used to urge health care professionals to consider a career in migrant health. In looking back on my own 30 years of involvement in caring for migrant and immigrant populations, I realize that the true description is both more complicated and more colorful than that.

As a family nurse practitioner (FNP) and certified nurse-midwife (CNM), I spent the first 20 years of my career providing direct care to patient populations that included significant numbers of immigrants who had come to my location—usually temporarily for work. For a decade since then I have had the opportunity to work on a national scale to provide support for other clinicians working in such settings.

Although I do not feel that advanced practice nurses (or any other health profession) are particularly well prepared for the task of caring for migrant patients, I do feel that we are well suited for the work. When faced with discussing pregnancy termination with a Haitian woman through an interpreter or developing a management plan for a woman who just had a cesarean section and was living in a car with her newborn and unemployed husband, I felt that I was at least as capable as any clinician to stumble through such interactions. The warmth and appreciation I received from patients was a bonus that made the work easier. A migrant patient never challenged my credentials or asked to be seen by "a real doctor." The women especially were visibly relieved to learn that they would be cared for by another woman.

I was fascinated by the challenge of addressing the impact on health of poverty, mobility, and difficult living and working conditions. Since farmworkers came to my northern location for only about 4 months of the year, I struggled with the desire to make a difference in a short period and with the frequent disappointment of not being able to follow through. Solving the puzzle of how to serve a transient and high-risk population in the context of the traditional health care system has been more than enough to keep me engaged for a lifetime.

FINDING MY WAY

As a freshly trained FNP, I approached the job market with the specific aims of getting some good primary care experience and making a living wage. I imposed a fairly significant limitation on my search by insisting on launching my career in the lovely but rural setting of central Pennsylvania.

In 1983, the role of the nurse practitioner (NP) was fairly new and especially unfamiliar where I lived. "Licensed Practical Nurse?" was often the question from those who were trying to understand. I had the added burden of explaining that I had followed an unconventional trajectory in receiving my NP education, first receiving a BA in psychology, then 10 years later entering a program that combined basic nursing and advanced practice, allowing me to emerge with an array of credentials: RN, FNP, and MS. I found potential employers in primary care practices, college health service, hospitals, and so on to be unimpressed by the initials after my name and gradually expanded the reach of my search to the nearest city, an hour away.

I was directed to a career in nursing by leanings toward both women's health and multicultural care. The former came from working for 5 years at the local family planning agency doing education and counseling during a time when the women's health movement was just that—a movement. As an outgrowth of the feminist revival of the 1970s, women demanded more information and involvement in their health care, resulting in dramatic changes in the availability of safe and reliable contraception, natural childbirth practices, and a stronger consumer voice in health care decision making. It was an exciting time to be involved.

My interest in other cultures was the result of a childhood of living and traveling in other countries, an experience that helped to shape my own personality and world view. It gave me an appreciation and interest in beliefs, practices, foods, and languages quite different from the homogenous and insulated complexion of the part of rural America I later chose as home.

Casting the wider net in my employment search resulted in two jobs—a full-time position with Planned Parenthood and a part-time seasonal post with the state migrant health program. Planned Parenthood rotated me among several sites, some as small as a staff of two (NP and receptionist), until I was charged with managing one of their small urban sites. The work was almost exclusively clinical—providing gynecological care to women—and included experienced NP colleagues, physicians who were supportive and appreciative of NPs, and an endless supply of patients. I learned efficiency, effective patient education, and how to leave judgment at the door. We were true experts in contraception, microscopy, sexually transmitted infections, and vaginitis, but were also able to delve into other conditions from anorexia to hypertension to shingles—as they arose.

> Lesson learned at Planned Parenthood: I was introduced here to the concept of charging for care based on the patient's ability to pay. It made perfect sense, since many of the women I cared for would not have been able to afford those services in a more conventional setting.

My first migrant health position was created for me after I convinced the program director that they needed an FNP. In retrospect, I'm certain that he responded more to my enthusiasm for the program than my NP skill set ("LPN?"). He was more accustomed to the yearly headache of finding capable staff willing to work odd hours seasonally than he was to having nurses call and beg to be hired. I was assigned to work four nights per week at three different evening clinic sites from June to November, while continuing to commute to the city for Planned Parenthood during the day. The schedule made me feel like something of a migrant myself but I recognized the opportunity as the career-defining experience that it was and jumped in. It was exhausting, exhilarating, and perfect. I saw a case of leprosy, spoke lots of Spanish, and learned that farmworkers were hidden throughout the hills and orchards around where I lived.

Acres of apples, peaches, and other fruits drew workers to this part of the world. Their work peaked in late summer and fall with the apple harvest, but also involved mowing, pruning, and other fieldwork from spring to fall. The packing houses employed seasonal labor to wash, sort, and pack produce for storage and shipping. In the 1980s, the migrant population represented a diverse mix of Latinos, Haitians, and African Americans. Most told us that they spent the winter months in Florida or Mexico, traveling northward each spring, stopping off to work in several locations as the growing season progressed. The workers were almost exclusively male, though some traveled with their families. Most lived in dormitory-style housing provided by their employers and had little contact with the local community. They depended on their crew leader for most of their needs outside the camp, including transportation and access to food, shopping, and health care.

AN INTRODUCTION TO MIGRANT HEALTH

A personal challenge in this initial migrant health position and in other settings early in my career was being in the awkward position of trying to promote the role of the NP to those I was working with while being utterly inexperienced and lacking in confidence. In other words, what would happen if I convinced them that I could take care of all those patients? What do you do for leprosy? As it turned out, there was plenty for everyone to do and each site was hosted by physicians who were delighted to have someone on board who shared their desire to serve this hard-working and underserved population. Without exception they shared interesting cases and patiently answered my questions.

Case 1

Melinda T. a patient whom I cared for in that first year, who helped me to take an early step up in my personal and professional awareness of the depth and complexity of health needs that are part of each exam room encounter. She presented for care at our migrant clinic and even in that diverse setting, she was unusual. She was White, for one thing, and English-speaking, though her partner was a Haitian farmworker. She was near 40, heavy, soft-spoken, and very pregnant. We provided care for the latter part of her pregnancy and one of the doctors attended the birth of her baby. I performed her postpartum examination and attempted to assess how well she was adjusting to motherhood. The baby was also seen and appeared to be doing well. Three weeks later she came in with severe headaches. She was hospitalized, diagnosed with cryptococcal meningitis, and died within days. This was the first AIDS case that any of us had been involved with.

One of the three sites was hosted by a private family practice group who had turned their office over to a migrant clinic in the evenings for a few years before I came along. This separate-but-equal approach worked well for them since the farmworkers did not want to miss work during daytime hours and their presence in the waiting room in the evening would not intimidate the more conventional private patients who preferred appointments during the day. A state health department grant supported a small ancillary staff of a nurse and van driver who visited the farms and orchards to perform outreach health status assessments, health education, and arranging appointments and transportation for our evening clinics. When the farmworker patients were brought in, we were able to provide state-of-the-art primary care, including examinations, lab testing, medications, and even referrals and inpatient care as needed.

As the weather turned rainy and cold and the last of the apples were picked, I knew I would miss this work and thought about going with the farmworkers to Florida or Texas for the winter. I also shamelessly urged the physicians I had worked with to think about how great it would be for them to have an FNP in their practice. One of them apparently agreed and several months later I was working full time in a small-town private practice and had cut my daily commute in half. I know now that my advocate was a physician named Ed. We had connected over our shared past experience of living in Latin America and an almost conspiratorial passion for serving the underserved. It was the beginning of a life-long professional partnership and eventually led to life partnership—he is now my husband.

Lesson learned at the migrant clinic: Find allies; the work is too big to do alone.

For the next 8 years I lived what felt like a double life, providing year-round care to a mostly White and insured local population, and every summer welcoming the diverse farmworkers to our evening clinics. I loved the work in both settings and honed my clinical skills, especially in the areas of pediatrics, gynecology, prenatal, and wellness care.

The arrangement evolved over time in both positive and negative directions. Another ally arrived on the scene—a socially conscious nurse with grant-writing skills. She managed to wrest funding for the migrant health program from the state so that we had more local control over the budget and decision making. We were able to obtain a small space and daytime clinician staffing to allow for more flexible appointment scheduling for migrant patients. Localized direction of the program expanded services and increased our visibility in the community.

THE LARGER MIGRANT HEALTH COMMUNITY

As I looked beyond the conservative and insulated local health care community for professional support, I involved myself in my state and national professional organizations. As advanced practice nurses struggled with finding recognition in the American health care system, I realized that migrant health might be a niche where we would not have to work so hard to be appreciated. I presented at national conferences about the multidisciplinary model we were using in our migrant program, including practice data that showed that the majority of care was being provided by nonphysicians.

Four years into this work, I attended my first national conference of other migrant health programs and a previously unknown world opened up for me. This community was not defined by one's profession, but by the population being served. Most were working, like me, in settings that were receiving specific federal funding to provide services to migrant farmworkers. Although the locations, crops, and growing seasons varied, we were all working with similar challenges and under the same restraints. By attending these gatherings regularly, I received an education from my peers on a wildly varied and wholly practical range of topics: cultural competence, treatment of tropical diseases, immigration policy, low-literacy patient education, outreach programs, dangers of pesticide exposure, and so forth.

A subgroup of the migrant health community—the Migrant Clinicians Network (MCN)—from then on became my professional home (and now employer!). It was an organization dedicated to providing resources for health care workers involved with caring for migrant patients.

SETTLING OUT

Case 2

> Isabel S. was a 16-year-old Mexican girl who had been in the United States for two months the first time I saw her. She was accompanied by Consuela S., the matriarch of a Mexican farmworker family that had lived in our area for many years and who were established patients of ours. Isabel and Consuela's teenaged son had wasted no time falling in love, getting pregnant, and deciding to get married. After performing a (positive!) pregnancy test and enrolling her for prenatal care, I advised her that she would be seeing the doctor at her next visit and would alternate appointments between him and me, as was our practice. As though she did not hear this, Consuela said that they were happy that Isabel would be able to see me because I was able to speak Spanish. I reminded her that the doctor also spoke Spanish. "But she doesn't want to see a man," was the response, accompanied by a smile and a huge bag of apples. So Isabel saw me for all of her prenatal care.

Our small town gradually experienced the phenomenon of "settling out" of some of the migrant population, as was occurring in farming communities across America in the 1980s and 1990s—as mobile workers found other more stable work opportunities, they and their families increasingly became year-round residents, working in factories, construction, and restaurants. Our year-round Latino population gradually grew. While this posed huge challenges to local schools, landlords, social services, and long-time community members, they were welcomed by their employers, many churches, and our small band of migrant health workers. Their appointments appeared increasingly on our daytime schedules as we managed their chronic illnesses and pregnancies. They were generally unable to access health care services otherwise due to language barriers; lack of insurance; and for those who were undocumented, inability to qualify for programs such as Medicaid.

I realize now that the erosion of the separate-but-equal approach to health care for the needy was taking place on a national scale and that transition was reflected in various developments in our community. For example, our local state health department services (immunizations, well child care, sexually transmitted disease [STD] clinics) were gradually dismantled and the hospital's Medicaid-only prenatal clinic became obsolete as reimbursement improved and physicians welcomed those patients into their practices.

Another more difficult trend was that while I found myself attending weddings and christenings in the growing Latino community, others in our practice became less supportive of hosting and working at the evening clinics in the office. The private practice had grown to the point that the physicians were tremendously busy with full-scope family practice, which at that time included on-call, inpatient care, and labor and delivery duties. Over time, the commitment of all but my greatest allies slipped away. Fortunately, our grant-writing colleague was more visionary and aware of the big-picture changes in the health care landscape than any of us. She recognized the greater need of the poor in the community and set her sights on obtaining federal funding to establish comprehensive care for *everyone* in the community—immigrants or fifth generation, White or not, insured or not.

BACK TO SCHOOL

New goals for my own professional development led me back to school. After working for several years in a family practice setting, my scope included taking care of children, adults, and pregnant women. I did teaching rounds in the hospital for all the new moms in the practice to review basics about infant care, breastfeeding, and postpartum issues and saw all of the newborns for their first office visit. As I gained confidence in my skills and appreciation for the continuity of care offered by the family practice model, I felt a desire to fill the critical missing link of attending births.

The Frontier School of Nursing and Midwifery offered a distance learning program that was a perfect fit for me. It built on the women's health experience I already had and added the perinatal skill set I was looking for, anchoring it to a solid knowledge base and abundant clinical experience.

Emerging from my midwifery training with even more initials after my name (CNM), I was well prepared to become one of the first clinicians to work at the fledgling federally funded community health center (CHC) that had come into being while I was away at school. Though much of the infancy of that organization was spent defining our vision, leadership, and our role in the medical community, there was no lack of patients. Spanish-speaking providers, a sliding fee scale, and evening hours attracted the uninsured and unattached, which included most of the Latino immigrants in the community. The poor appreciated the dignity of feeling welcomed by an organization that offered the care they needed for themselves and their families. I shared their sense of coming home, knowing that my work was no longer compartmentalized based on who the patient was that I was taking care of.

THE COMMUNITY HEALTH CENTER EXPERIENCE

Case 3

> Since farmworkers typically came to our area only during the growing season, it was rare that I would care for a migrant woman through her entire pregnancy. Liliana was one of those women who came early in her pregnancy and had not had any prenatal care. This was her seventh pregnancy, and during her health history she reported that all of her six children had been born at home in Mexico without any difficulties. When we proceeded to her examination she told me matter-of-factly that she had never had a pelvic exam before.

In addition to expanding comprehensive primary care services to anyone regardless of his or her ability to pay, our CHC grant included funds earmarked specifically to continue the migrant health program. The organization supported outreach to the farmworker camps as we had done in the past, but we were able to accommodate those patients into the health center schedule whenever it worked for *them.* The program required adding a few seasonal employees who performed most of the fieldwork locating workers on farms or in motels, taking health histories, performing basic health screenings and education, registering them for services, and arranging appointments as needed. My role in the migrant program continued to be seeing patients for primary care consultations: men with high blood pressure, sore muscles, or worried about sexually transmitted infections (STIs); children for vaccinations and coughs; and, my favorite, the women.

Soon after the CHC opened its doors, a factory that makes plastic flower pots moved to our community from New Jersey, bringing along most of its nearly 500 Guatemalan employees (and their families)—an overnight transformation for our small town.

I had a front-row seat in observing an organization in constant transition over the next several years. We added staff and expanded services to include dental, social work, counseling, pharmacy, and interpretation services. We added additional sites and built a beautiful facility to accommodate the burgeoning demand. As an FNP/CNM ("family nurse-midwife") I was able to see a broad scope of patients and developed my own patient case load, many of whom were Spanish-speaking immigrant families.

I felt that I was finally working in a truly multidisciplinary setting that respected the contribution of each member of the team. In retrospect, I can identify several possible explanations for the success of that team:

- I was married by then to the medical director who had been thoroughly brainwashed on the subject of collaborative multidisciplinary care.
- We were all employees and on salary, so that no one was making money off of someone else's work.
- The general term of "practitioner" was used to refer to physicians, NPs, CNMs, and physician assistants, and collective groans were heard in response to the terms "mid-level providers" or " physician extenders." We all participated in peer review of each other, used the same clinical guidelines, and had our own patient panels.
- Most of our physician recruits came straight from residency, had some experience working with multidisciplinary teams, and were more open to collaborative practice.
- We were, for the most part, all motivated by the "mission" of working at a CHC and working for the underserved, meaning that egos were less involved.

I wanted to contribute to the success of the organization by providing quality care, having satisfied patients, and being efficient. I took on some administrative duties and participated in enough quality management, performance improvement, and clinical management activities to appreciate the big picture of keeping a health center viable. Open communication from leadership allowed me to understand the simple need to balance the expense of clinician salaries with revenue generated by patient visits and services, though productivity was inevitably an area of friction between those in management and those providing patient care. The motivation to make it all work sustained me through many years of demanding patient appointment schedules, on-call hours, and attending births at the hospital day and night.

¿Habla español?

My engagement with the immigrant population extended beyond the health center and included activities such as organizing a women's health group for Spanish-speaking women to talk about various issues, teaching Spanish childbirth classes, supporting the development of a community Hispanic center, and providing short-term housing for refugees. All of it deepened my understanding and appreciation of the Latino culture and broadened my language skills.

When seeing patients I usually worked without an interpreter, calling for help when I wanted to ensure informed consent for a procedure or when a visit took on the flavor of a counseling session and I knew I could not negotiate the nuances of a complex psychological situation. A need for greater confidence in my language skills took me on multiple 2- or 3-week trips to Guatemala for language school. There came a point, however, when I realized that language skill does not equal cultural competence. As I got to know my patients and their trust grew, some of the stories that I heard included descriptions of mystical connections between an emotional trauma and a physical symptom (*susto*), spells and curses, herbal cures, and probably some other things that I never did understand. I found myself being faced with disconnects and questions that I couldn't reconcile. How can a woman leave her children behind to come to the United States and work in a factory or a packing house? Why is it apparently so unimportant to keep appointments for prenatal visits? Does everyone really buy in to that whole machismo deal? And the biggest question: How bad was the life left behind that this is an improvement?

BEYOND THE BORDER

While I had no intention of leaving my job, I wanted to learn more about where my patients had come from. I told the Guatemalans that I wanted to visit their country to see if it was as lovely as its people. It was. Language school in Antigua was a perfect place to start—with one-on-one language instruction, living with a local family, and visiting cultural and historical sights.

The next step was to figure out a way to provide health care in Central America in a way that would make me feel less like a tourist and not require me to leave my life and work behind. An NP friend and I took a trip to Nicaragua under the care of a sister-cities program to learn about the health care system there. We were taken to rural clinics, urban hospitals, medical and nursing schools, grassroots health education programs, and people's homes. The crushing poverty and unlimited need were offset by the contagious energy and spirit driving every organization that we visited.

Ed and I later found our way to an organization working in Honduras that provided us with the opportunity to do meaningful work on a short-term basis. Shoulder to Shoulder, like many nongovernmental organizations (NGOs), supports the development of health care services in a small corner of the world and welcomes volunteer clinicians to help in providing those services. Unlike many NGOs, however, they work in a true partnership with their host communities while the visiting volunteers simply augment the full-time presence of local clinic staff. The organization has a long history of providing a learning environment for American medical and nursing students that is often a life-changing experience.

While my personal goal in Honduras was to shed light on my understanding of the migrant experience, it was impossible not to respond to the intense needs there. Over time, I took at least 20 trips to various parts of Honduras, mostly to rural isolated areas of intense poverty, sleeping in schools and dormitories and eating beans and tortillas. After having my fill of working in makeshift clinics with endless lines of patients and few medications and supplies, I looked for a way to make a more satisfying—and hopefully more sustainable—contribution. I naturally gravitated toward women's health and made connections with the community-based *parteras* (midwives) whenever possible. With each meeting there was an instant connection when I told them that I too was a midwife. In one such conversation I asked what they did when complications arise during birth, and one of the *parteras* said that she always felt the presence on her shoulder of an angel watching over her and the mother. In spite of our drastically different practice settings I acknowledged that the same midwife angel had helped me out too.

To learn more about their work I did a formal survey of 39 *parteras* in the region and learned that they attended most of the births in their villages (in the women's homes), their training and skills were rudimentary, and, despite performing a critical service, they functioned without any official position in the health care system. In a discussion of their training needs, one of them blurted out, "Teach us something now!" so I did an impromptu lesson on calculating due dates.

The passionate plea for more education was loud and clear, prompting my own adventure in popular education methodology and cultural competence. I learned in working with these traditional midwives that rather than low-literacy teaching methods, it was best to use "no-literacy" approaches. I learned the hard way that even two-dimensional drawings could be difficult for some of the women to "read." With the help of the Hesperian Health Guides (*Where Women*

Have No Doctor, A Book for Midwives, and *Helping Health Workers Learn*), I developed teaching units that relied on local resources props, people, and stories, and emphasized hands on practice of skills. A pregnant woman from the community was a model for teaching Leopold's maneuvers to a small group. Various vegetables and fruits were used to demonstrate measurement of fundal height. Cultural awareness was integrated into this approach in that participants were encouraged to share their experiences and knowledge, and nonharmful traditional practices were embraced.

More than any other experience, my work with *parteras* in this safe and empowering learning environment provided me with insights that helped me to understand my immigrant patients at home. I realized that the lack of trust in doctors and the health care system in general was a result of disrespectful treatment and discouraging results of care received in their home countries; that what seemed like passivity about health care issues was really a faith-based acceptance of God's intentions (*fatalismo*); and that the reliance on an unlimited range of folk practices and beliefs *(creencias)* was widespread. Most of all, it confirmed a lesson I continue to learn; that is, little is accomplished in the absence of a trusting relationship (*confianza*).

MIGRANT CLINICIANS NETWORK

After 18 years of working in the Pennsylvania migrant health program, my family moved to a relatively affluent university town that had hardly any migrant farmworkers at all. This change of venue brought about a dramatic change in my professional life as well, as I moved away from full-time clinical work and began to work for the Migrant Clinicians Network (MCN). For 4 years I managed a program for MCN that was a perfect fit for me—a practicum in migrant health for newly graduated clinicians. It involved selecting, placing, and mentoring new NPs, CNMs, physician assistants, and dental hygienists in migrant health programs for a 4-month supervised work experience. It was an ideal opportunity to promote the contributions of these professions and multidisciplinary care, to introduce promising clinicians to the world of migrant health, and to learn about migrant and community health centers around the country.

Since then I have provided clinical input for a variety of MCN programs and activities—family violence prevention, environmental and occupational health, case management of mobile patients, and clinician education. Most of that work has involved direct interaction with people who are caring for migrant patients. Presentations at conferences, training health promoters, and responding to requests from the field for clinical support are typical activities.

While my past clinical practice experience informs every bit of this work, it has required the development of an entirely new set of skills, including public speaking, research, writing, managing program expenses, and evaluation of program outcomes. Working from a home office also means embracing the technology that makes it possible to work with people in five other locations and across three time zones. E-mail, conference calls with desktop sharing, instant messaging, and a shared server for document storage and data entry are all tools of the trade. Communication with a far-flung constituency requires an appreciation of the power of a website, photographs, and social media. And who knew that PowerPoint was an art form? The flexibility offered by a home-based office balanced with the demands of frequent travel away from home results in a work life that is never predictable or boring.

RETROSPECTIVE: THREE DECADES LATER

From the vantage point of someone who is in "late career," it is gratifying to recognize that what has felt at times to be a winding road has been held together by the common thread of providing health care service to migrants and immigrants. The profession of nursing armed me with an array of practical skills and a holistic philosophy of care that became my admission ticket into a world I would not otherwise have been able to enter. I have been so fortunate to have had work that allowed me to peer into the shadows of inequity and injustice in the world and in doing so to find a way to contribute to improving the lives of those I have served.

REFERENCES

Hesperian Health Guides. Retrieved from www.hesperian.org
Migrant Clinicians Network. Retrieved from www.migrantclinician.org
Migrant and Community Health Centers. Retrieved from http://bphc.hrsa.gov
Shoulder to Shoulder. Retrieved from www.shouldertoshoulder.org

6

Therapeutic Communication

Bridging Cultural and Language Differences

CHRISTINA MARTINEZ KIM

Editor's Note: As a student, Christina Martinez Kim was drawn to psychiatric-mental health nursing. She also had a strong desire to work globally but wasn't sure psych-mental health offered the appropriate skill set to bridge the cultural and language barriers she would encounter. Christina recognizes that therapeutic communication can be difficult to establish in emotionally charged situations where we do not share a common language or life experience with our patients. However, she makes a compelling argument that there is much to be shared in the human experience even when spoken communication is limited.

At an early age, I had a visceral affinity for Mother Teresa's work in the slums of Calcutta among the untouchables. I saw TV clips of the hands-on, healing work she and other sisters did, washing feet, bandaging wounds, feeding orphans. They were fighting against disparity, injustice, marginalization, and death. It's no wonder that at age 9 I told my dad I wanted to become a nun.

TV also introduced me to the movie *El Norte*—in which a brother and sister fleeing genocide in Guatemala cross the United States–Mexico border, only to have the sister die from a rat bite. I was struck by the loss and angry at what I knew was a preventable death. My father tried to console me, saying "life is not fair." I resisted the idea, believing that just because life is not fair it doesn't mean I can't do something about it. If anything, it was a chance to discover my agency. A lifelong desire to work with and for the "other" was effectively seeded.

Another major factor, behind my choice of profession, is my minority status. I am a fourth-generation Mexican American, born to Mexican-American parents, who themselves didn't speak much Spanish as kids and never taught it to me. I grew up in a small town in Arizona, a town my family had helped pioneer decades before I was born. Even so, there were plenty of times I felt out of place. The dominant culture and my peers didn't have relatives who spoke Spanish at family events. They didn't have 50 first cousins. They didn't eat menudo and tamales, have piñatas at their birthday parties, or have brown skin and darker features.

NURSING

After graduation from college, I worked in a public health research lab. My colleagues were great, the work was interesting, I was salaried, but I realized I didn't want to do research. I realized that what I missed was dealing with people rather than samples. Recognizing that desire is what led me to nursing.

I saw how in demand nurses were at the time and the various jobs they held. I liked the flexibility of nursing and the promise to always have a job. Nursing also seemed to reflect the mission of Mother Teresa, which had inspired me as a child. Once in a nursing program, my only problem was my genuine like for all my rotations without a commitment to any one specialty area. I do remember though that the one rotation that spoke to me most was psychiatry. I'd been assigned to an inpatient mental health crisis unit and the experience was a mix of scary, exciting, foreign, and enticing. I was fascinated by the intricacy of the mind–body intersection and how horribly wrong things could get with seemingly small perturbations. Life felt very fragile.

While I was excited by the work and wanted to know more, I felt that nursing school discouraged any consideration of a career in psychiatric nursing. A mentor shared a comment by one of her advisors years ago that "only the bad nurses go into psychiatry."

I felt a strong desire to work with vulnerable populations in global environments, if possible. This desire is probably what clinched my choice of mental health despite the misgivings raised during nursing school. As I put out feelers to solicit support—rather than advice—I attended a mission conference at my church. The speakers were medical doctors who had worked in international settings serving the poorest, sickest, and most vulnerable populations imaginable.

In response to my questions, one of the speakers revealed that she had considered a residency in psychiatry years earlier. What changed her mind, however, was the complexity of providing psychiatric care across cultural and language barriers.

I knew I wanted to work globally. However, without an inherent understanding of the cultural context underlying mental health and the ability to communicate effectively in a patient's language, how could I expect to forge a therapeutic relationship within which to establish trust and create hope? I had no clear response to these questions so I shelved the thought of pursuing an advanced nursing degree in mental health—at least for the time being.

BOSTON

After relocating to Boston with my husband shortly after graduation, I interviewed at the Brigham and Women's Hospital for a staff nurse position. The hospital was adjacent to Harvard's medical campus and the Dana-Farber Cancer Institute. I was in Paul Farmer and Jim Kim territory, both of whom who I greatly admired. I had read Tracy Kidder's *Mountains Beyond Mountains*, which chronicles the genesis of the Boston-based Partners in Health and its remarkable work in Haiti. When the hospital offered me a position, I didn't hesitate.

My introduction to nursing at Brigham was tough. In retrospect, I think this is the case for most new nurses regardless of where they work. The rotating shifts and an inability to sleep for more than 4 to 5 hours during the day when I was on nights were hard. The complexity and diversity of patients I encountered was hard. But mostly it was hard because Brigham didn't have a dedicated psychiatric floor.

A common occurrence was the admission of patients with psychiatric needs in addition to medical comorbidities. It was a salient moment when I realized how important knowledge of psychiatry was. I cared for patients who had anxiety as a consequence of hospitalization, depression due to chronic illness, persons suffering from acute delirium, as well as someone with dementia secondary to HIV. I still remember the patient who suffered a stroke after years of cocaine use, a young patient who was having an adjustment reaction after suffering a pulmonary embolus, and the patient deemed, after a psych consult, to be malingering and not acutely psychotic. It was on-the-ground training and not something I'd expected. Though I was still unsure of a specialty, I decided to go back to school to become a nurse practitioner. I wanted to attend my alma mater, and so back to North Carolina we went.

GLOBAL IS LOCAL

While preparing for graduate school, I accepted a job at a local community health center that serves a predominance of Latino immigrants. The opportunity to work with low-resourced patients, many of whom were not native English speakers, was a big draw. My Spanish was not strong and I valued the opportunity to hone my language skills.

It was my responsibility to handle incoming calls and to make assessments over the phone or in person, if someone came to the clinic sans appointment. Assessments varied between giving advice for symptomatic relief of diarrhea to ruling out possible stroke and the need to send someone to the emergency department. Many of the assessments were conducted in Spanish, over the phone, which made things more complicated.

Another challenge was the low level of health literacy of many clinic patients. My cobbled form of Spanish probably helped in this department. I didn't know the medical terminology for certain symptoms and disorders, so I had to keep explanations simple and free of medical jargon. My lack of technical vocabulary and the need to come up with longish explanations along with difficulty conjugating verbs all worked together to give me frequent headaches. Though patients were gracious and patient, there were times I had to check and recheck that what I'd heard was correct and what I meant to say was actually what was understood. All this offered me a small glimpse into the frustration and vulnerability patients often feel, surrounded by persons who do not speak their native tongue.

It's important to note that these patients, though many of them spoke Spanish, were from several countries spanning South and Central America as well as Mexico. This diversity reflected different cultures, different idioms, different accents, and sometimes different words to express the same thing or idea. One might think the Spanish language is the same the world over. There are variations, just as there are with English across regions of the United States and the United Kingdom.

The community health center is where my formal training connected with my desire to work with and for the underdog in a global environment while still working locally. For me "global" really had become "local." I was paid to do a job that was fulfilling and challenging. I was living in a community just a couple miles from the University of North Carolina campus and working with patients from all around the world. As a nursing student, I wouldn't have guessed this was possible, but it was happening and I hadn't stepped out of North Carolina to do it. The world had become smaller, as evidenced by the commonality of basic human emotions and needs.

Along the way, I discovered the propensity to be a listener. I recognized there was more in common between people than in what separates us. I trusted that I could learn how to effectively bridge cultural and language barriers. I'd already made great progress in developing those skills while working locally. Why couldn't I become prepared to work in an international setting, as well? It was a leap of faith, but in the end, I thought I'd be doing myself a disservice if I didn't at least try. So, after a year back in North Carolina, I submitted my application to graduate school—in mental health.

GHANA

It was my husband who took us to Ghana—a West African country I had barely heard of before he was offered a job. We had always talked about living and working abroad, but the opportunity to do so came much sooner than anticipated. Over the course of 4 weeks, he had two international interviews, received a solid job offer, and began making plans to relocate us. I was in the middle of my master's program and needed to complete two clinical rotations before I could join him. Our 4-month separation was not pleasant. However, my husband's physical presence in Ghana turned out to be essential in completing the steps required for me to join him while still being able to finish my program. I had received blessings for my proposal from my academic advisor as well as the director of the master's program. This in and of itself was big. What's more, I'd been given permission to take my remaining courses online and to participate in class discussions via Skype.

My husband's task was to search for an appropriate psychiatry preceptor, which I needed to complete my capstone course while in Ghana. This was a big hurdle. The preceptor had to meet specific criteria to be eligible—namely she or he had to be a psychiatric nurse practitioner or a psychiatrist who worked onsite at a mental health facility. Finding such a person could be very difficult because—at the time—there were only about 15 psychiatrists in the entire country for a population of roughly 24 million. Most of the psychiatrists, fortunately, were based in the capital, Accra, where we'd be living. My husband's coworkers suggested he contact the Medical Director of the Accra Psychiatric Hospital (APH), Dr. Akwasi Osei, who was also the chief psychiatrist of Ghana Health Service, the country's national health system.

Dr. Osei was probably bemused by my husband, a large Asian man, asking if he would precept his Mexican-American wife, a nurse practitioner student, planning to finish her final practicum in Ghana. Fortunately, he agreed to precept me at the Accra Psychiatric Hospital, and I was on my way to Ghana.

Getting Started

Prior to leaving for Ghana, I did some research about the APH and mental health care in Ghana. In one article, I found disturbing information about a nurse at the hospital who had been assaulted and another who had been killed. A second article mentioned the proposed Mental Health Reform Bill. Other than those two reports, I had little to go on. I realized that once again I was making a leap of faith.

My first days at the hospital were a bit of blur. I recall meeting the Director of Nursing, Mr. Anyetei, as well as several staff nurses with names like Doris, Florence, Agnes, and Gifty. In those first few days, I also met a couple psychiatrists, a medical resident finishing her psychiatric rotation, and a psychiatric physician's assistant.

Although it was clear that Dr. Osei would be my preceptor, there was some confusion over what I could and would actually do at the hospital. Nurse practitioners do not exist in Ghana, though psychiatric physician assistants do. As such, when I was introduced, people often missed the fact I was a master's student who would eventually prescribe psychotropics.

Most people seemed more comfortable calling me a nurse, though in practice I soon would have responsibilities more akin to the psychiatric prescribers. For this reason as well as some uncertainty about what to do with me, I was given over to the Director of Nursing. This plan gave me the opportunity to get to know the various hospital wards and to see firsthand the work done primarily by nurses.

My start date at APH coincided with nursing students from a local public university beginning their psychiatric rotation. I saw varied responses as some of them kept themselves to the perimeter away from patients and staff, whereas others were in the thick of the action talking with patients and performing various nurse tasks. I saw some of them tear up at the conditions of the hospital and the needs of the patients.

What was most memorable, however, were the patients themselves and the hospital. I should inject here that I have very little firsthand knowledge of what psychiatric institutions look like, how they feel and operate. When I was a nursing student I toured Dorothea Dix Hospital in North Carolina for a day and got a basic, quick introduction to institutionalized mental health care. Other than that, I had never spent time in a long-term psychiatric care facility.

The Hospital

What I saw at the APH was what I imagined mental institutions were like 100 years ago, plus electricity. In fairness, the APH was never planned to be what it had become, the largest psychiatric institution in West Africa. It was born out of the need to house persons with mental health disorders who had been rounded up by local police. It was designed with open courtyards and open trenches to carry away sewage. These open trenches were used as latrines by male patients on some of the locked wards. Public urination in Ghana is common so its extension to the hospital might not have been regarded as abnormal by nationals. In my mind's eye, however, urinating in broad daylight on a locked ward somehow heightened the depravity of the situation.

The hospital had grown to accommodate over 1,000 patients, though the facility had only 600 beds. Because there were too few beds, rolled up mats and foam pads came out at night. A pervasive smell of rot, waste, and lots of flies made eating my peanut butter and jelly sandwiches difficult the first week. The campus included several wards—some locked and others more porous.

The entire campus was closed with a guard at the main gate topped with rolled barbwire. Patients who roamed the campus freely or were sent to fetch water and meals greeted me. One patient made an announcement of my arrival to the ward exclaiming, "There's somebody from America, thank God!" On a ward primarily for children with developmental disabilities, a young boy, maybe 7 or 8 years old, constantly touched my arms and hair signaling he wanted to be picked up.

The Wards

I found each ward at APH had its own flavor, with varying resources and expectations. One female ward kept a low census of about 20 women. It was not locked, and though there were inmates, that is, patients, who liked to abscond they simply didn't. Maybe it was the debilitating psychosis that had brought them to the hospital, maybe it was the nurses' station in the center of the courtyard, or the reality of not having anywhere else to go. There were few formalized activities, although there was some structure in morning singing, taking of meds, and patients going for treatment including electroconvulsive therapy (ECT).

Another ward—a men's locked ward for persons with psychosis—had a very different feel. There was a locked antechamber to help prevent escape, though inmates frequently eloped when let off premises with family members. Involuntary commitment was common. The majority of inpatients were brought in as a last resort, having already gone to local healers and shamans. By the time they got to the hospital, many were actively psychotic, manic, or physically aggressive.

On one male ward, I was told patients experiencing psychosis had torn down screening intended to prevent the entry of mosquitos. The ward had long dormitories exposed to the elements with tin roofs to offer some protection. Sleeping quarters were locked at approximately 6:30 p.m. and reopened in the morning at 6:00 a.m. Patients were confined to small spaces with little to no protection from disease-bearing vectors including malaria-carrying mosquitos. All that remained was a wire grid effective only for keeping patients inside the dorms. Cisterns were kept in the dorms for urination and defecation. Not surprisingly, malaria and tuberculosis were common. These conditions were largely the result of running a hospital well over capacity—not out of choice—but rather necessity.

Managing Care

With a census of well over 1,000 and fewer than four psychiatric prescribers working on any given day, there was little rounding done on the wards by the admitting staff. I had just completed a rotation in the States where each patient was seen and interviewed by the attending psychiatrist for at least 10 minutes each day, and sometimes more frequently. More often than not, the patient was also seen by a medical resident, perhaps a medical student, a psychologist(s) for individual and/or group therapy, all in addition to the assigned psychiatric nurse. Unfortunately at the APH, the psychiatric prescribers had to prioritize their interventions and were primarily only able to see outpatients, persons who were formerly hospitalized, or persons whose decline had been caught and treated before becoming more severe.

Outpatient appointments weren't really appointments. Patients simply showed up in the morning and waited to see their provider—who might or might not be there. Often, it was the prescriber's nurse who kept the patients updated and arranged for them to see a different provider if they had traveled a long distance or were acutely ill. A 5-minute medication check was the only feasible way to meet the demands of large numbers of patients who had been waiting for hours to have their medications renewed.

I remember working with a psychiatrist who saw 35 to 40 patients in the course of a 5-hour day. He did this four to five times a week. With such a caseload, it was nearly impossible for him to round on patients on the wards. Besides, the outpatient clinic was a lot less depressing than the wards. One psychiatrist told me he avoided one of the wards, in particular, because walking through it brought him to tears.

The staff at the APH had to accept limitations, ones often outside their control. They had chosen a career in mental health in order to make a difference, but the obstacles to providing care were many.

Medications

The inconsistent supply of medications was a significant barrier to adequate care. One day there might be an antipsychotic or anticonvulsant available free of charge, as they were covered by the national health program for hospital patients. The next day could turn up a shortage or complete absence of medication. One young nurse dealt with this problem by opting to switch one antidepressant for another when the prescribed med ran out. He didn't consult with the prescriber or compare dosage equivalencies. Medication errors were not uncommon.

The system for dispensing meds consisted of a wooden board with cutouts to hold small glass vials. A long piece of masking tape ran along the bottom of each row of vials and numbers were written on the tape, corresponding to patient ID numbers. Patients were responsible for remembering their identifying numbers. They queued up each day to get their meds, but understandably some got their IDs wrong or remembered an ID from a prior admission. This led to a patient taking someone else's meds or missing meds altogether. I am not sure which was worse. I never did see the five rights of medication administration while at the APH.

Stigma

Stigma was another barrier to care. A psychiatric nurse at the hospital confided she didn't usually tell family members where she worked; only that she was a nurse. She felt if it got out she was caring for "mad" people she'd catch sidelong glances, be reprimanded, or be suspected of being "mad" herself.

Stigma also led to patients being abandoned at the hospital, long after recovery. This had become so common that the hospital started collecting a fee from each patient upon admission. The money was used to fuel a bus once a month to return patients to their villages. Mental illness caused such shame and/or burden among family members that some were actively tricked into coming to Accra to collect a patient at the hospital. Staff recounted one occasion when a family was informed of a patient's death. The patient's family promptly traveled to Accra to collect a body, only to find their relative was alive and well, and ready to go home with them.

Advocacy

Lack of personnel translated into variable care for the patients. Some wards were better staffed, with five or more nurses for 20 patients, whereas other wards had only a few nurses to care for nearly 200 patients. This discrepancy affected patient length of stay, as it was the nurses who decided when a patient was ready for discharge. They were the ones who brought a patient's chart to the psychiatric prescriber for review and possible discharge.

I spent a good deal of time with a female patient, D, who had been admitted for a psychotic break late in life. When I first met her, she'd been on the ward for a few weeks. She was faithfully taking her medication and the psychosis had remitted; she was no longer endorsing paranoid delusions. My question then became, "Why is she still here?" She had resources, a family member involved in her care, and adequate finances to support herself though she was unemployed. These circumstances were rare and together they poised the patient for a smooth transition back into the community. She wanted to get out of the hospital, but her chart hadn't been brought before one of the prescribers, so she was stuck.

I remember feeling frustrated and uncertain at the same time with D's case. I was constantly reminded of being an obroni, a foreigner. One time a nurse reprimanded a fellow nurse for interrupting our conversation, asking the question, "Can't you see I'm talking to a White lady?" Remember I am Mexican American and brown. I have brown hair, brown eyes, and I have never been mistaken for a "White lady" in America.

I had a difficult time formulating a plan of action. If I complained about the unfairness of denying someone her rights, I probably would have been shut out in a polite, but definite way. I was a guest at the hospital and a foreigner to Ghana. I hadn't grown up there or had a chance to learn the culture. I'd barely arrived. Yet, I felt confronted with fundamental ethical questions. Who was I to question the status quo? Did I believe people had basic rights regardless of where they were physically located? Did I really believe people with severe and persistent mental illness could make decisions on their own behalf? Or was treatment more relative, specific to local customs and traditions? Is it just another of way of saying, "That's the way we do it here?"

I reaffirmed my philosophy, partly informed by egalitarian standards I grew up with in America, largely informed by my Christian faith. Yes, there are basic rights for all human beings regardless of gender, illness, and country of origin. There was a right and a wrong and what I was seeing was definitely wrong. I wanted to be heard and to engage in a discussion rather than shove my ideas at people; knowing that to do so might lead to change but, most likely, only temporarily. I hoped that leading by example might work and so I advocated for a handful of patients. I brought their paper charts before the prescribers. I suggested medication changes to decrease side effects that would make anyone want to stop taking their medication cold turkey.

This tactic worked for D. I saw her discharged home on an atypical antipsychotic and arranged for outpatient follow-up at the hospital. Unfortunately, it didn't work for another patient. After 3 months of involuntary commitment and many rounds of electroconvulsive therapy, she simply walked out of the hospital. She'd gone out to buy food for other patients and never returned. I had worked it out for her admitting psychiatrist to evaluate her on the ward hoping for discharge, but I heard he never came.

Though my time at the hospital was rich and offered much for personal reflection, I wish I could report that my presence encouraged many changes. However, to be honest, I doubt that is the case. After 1 year, my husband and I moved back to North Carolina. A new chapter in my nursing career was about to begin.

EL FUTURO

My experiences in Ghana had answered some questions about the efficacy of mental health skills in global settings but it raised others. However, I returned home with a renewed sense of purpose regarding the importance of developing therapeutic relationships that are effective across cultural and language barriers.

In thinking about where I would like to work next, I immediately thought of El Futuro, a nonprofit mental health agency, where I had interned as a graduate student. The three semesters I spent working with the El Futuro staff and patients were incredible. I experienced the magic I had seen as a nursing student on the psychiatric crisis unit. Patients and staff at El Futuro were receptive, encouraging, and gracious. I felt kinship with the agency's mission to provide mental health care to the local Spanish-speaking community.

My new position was interesting because I was asked to do therapy exclusively. I thoroughly enjoyed therapy, but felt it was a weaker aspect of my practice. Should I accept a therapy position without more formal training? Would I lose my knowledge of psychopharmacology? I took the job hoping the experience in psychotherapy would round out my practice.

I grew in ways I didn't foresee. I heard many stories of endurance and fortitude that caused me to feel embarrassed that I had ever complained about anything. In session, it was as though a veil was lifted, pretenses fell away, and deep issues remained awaiting examination, analysis, change. I had to learn to be comfortable with silence, to let people problem solve for themselves, and to not assume I had the answer. All of this had to be done in a setting where the majority of patients were recent immigrants to the United States who brought to our encounters a wealth of life experience unfamiliar to me. It was a dance—an improvised one at that.

The conclusion of my first year at El Futuro offered an opportunity to reflect on my practice. I was able to reexamine my call to the profession. Was I doing what I dreamed I would be doing when I chose nursing? Had I enhanced my therapeutic communication skills sufficiently to bridge cultural and language barriers? If so, was I using those skills to serve the most vulnerable in society to right the injustices of this world?

Different days lead to different responses to each of these questions. I am now confident that psychiatric-mental health nurse practitioners bring a unique skill set to the well-being of patients both at home and abroad. I have come full circle since my days at the community health center, with an even greater appreciation for the concept that "global is local" and for my place in this world and the contributions I make to it.

7

Hope for a Changing System

Experiences of a Haitian Colleague

NAOMIE MARCELIN

Editor's Note: Naomie Marcelin is a Haitian nurse working for Zanmi Lasante in Haiti, which is a sister organization to Partners in Health cofounded by Dr. Paul Farmer. Naomie's voice represents that of the community she serves. She has worked for years with colleagues represented by contributors to this collection. I asked her describe what she believes Americans and Europeans working in Haiti need to know. She does so with humor and tact. Her narrative represents a nice point/counterpoint to those of several other authors.

I am a Haitian nurse who graduated from the national school in Port-au-Prince in 2002. I am from a family of five children: three girls and two boys. I lost one of my sisters in the earthquake of January 12, 2010. I am still single with no children and my family thinks that's because I've already given my heart to my profession. I always laugh at that joke.

I don't have an exciting story to share or something that everyone can be amazed at. I am a regular nurse who's working every day to help people in my country. Could I say that I am special because of my work? The answer could be yes and no. Every day, nurses around the world are doing the same things that I do to help my patients and contribute to changing the system in my country. Nursing care makes me and my work special and my satisfaction in being a nurse is the smile of my patients and their families. My story is not fiction and cannot make a reader dream. But I have had many wonderful experiences in my career—some sad and some unexpected—that strengthen and reinforce my commitment to being good at what I do and to share a part of it with you.

BECOMING A NURSE

Being able to study in the university in Haiti can be challenging for many students. The number of students graduating from high school is higher than the capacity of our universities. Students face two decisions: to be accepted into a university and to think about the type of job they can find after years of study. This reality puts them in a situation where they have to figure out how to find a job to support their family instead of choosing a career they really love.

Unfortunately, some nurses who don't like the profession fall into this category: "they went to nursing school because it's one of the professions in Haiti where finding a job is less difficult, not because they like it." Explaining this concept to foreign nurses and doctors that I've collaborated with is difficult.

When I started nursing school I was in that category: I enrolled in nursing after the completion of 7 years of high school, not because I loved it nor for the purpose of getting a job, but rather to please a good friend of mine who is a nurse. I've promised her I would take the qualifying exam for the national university—which I did and passed. However, my dream was to be a pediatrician because I love children, not to become a nurse.

AN UNFORGETABLE EXPERIENCE

A bad experience as a student changed my life forever. During one of my clinical rotations, I was mad when I found one of my patients lying in bed covered in feces. She was in a deplorable state of health. She couldn't move or talk and her prognosis was bad. Her eyes were closed but she was responsive to pain stimulation.

I was just a student. There was a lot I didn't understand yet and was not ready for, but I did understand that the patient needed my assistance. She needed to be washed and cleaned. My nursing colleagues were sitting in their office—laughing about a story—probably more important than their work and their patient's well-being, I suppose. I went to them and explained the situation and asked for assistance. None of them were willing to help. That revolted me so I asked another student nurse to help me. Finally the other student and I managed to bathe the patient and the result was satisfactory. After our care, the patient opened her eyes. She looked at me, smiled, turned her head to the side, and died. Our resuscitation attempts were not successful. It was my first death and I cried a lot.

After that experience I understood that nobody can be a good nurse if it's not from the heart. I embraced the profession and promised myself—in memory of that patient—to always do my best in taking care of all my patients.

A CHANCE TO LEARN FROM OTHERS

A wonderful part of my career has been the chance to learn from different kinds of people and cultures: nurses and doctors from different nursing and medical schools in Haiti as well as nurses and doctors from foreign countries. This variety of culture can make work partly difficult, partly exciting, and be a wonderful benefit.

The exciting and beneficial part results from working with nurses and doctors who have showed me that work can be done differently. Work as a nurse is not only coming to work, reading medical orders, giving medicine, and going home. It also requires understanding the illness and the patient. Ask yourself, "What is going on with my patient? What can I do to address the situation? How can I better help my patient?" As nursing students we learned how to make a plan of care for each patient—a practice we seem to lose as we start working professionally, unfortunately. Foreign nurses revived in me a taste for learning and asking questions. Why do we give this medication and not the other one? Why do we decrease the dose for this patient? Those are fundamental questions that some Haitian nurses don't ask anymore because they have a ton of work to do and don't have time to pay attention to understanding what they do. I've learned from foreign nurses how evidence-based practice is critical and that the best way to help your patient is to understand what is going on and why I do what I do. The more you understand, the more you know how important it is to give the medication on time, to pay attention to a patient's diet, intake and output, to check his weight and height, to take his blood pressure, and evaluate his heart rate before administering certain kinds of medication.

HAITIAN PEOPLE ARE NOT LIKE AFRICAN PEOPLE!

On the other hand, it is difficult and challenging to observe that cultural approaches are often misunderstood or forgotten by the foreign nurses. It can be really challenging to make them understand that what works perfectly in hospitals in their country don't necessarily fit with Haiti's reality. It's also important to recognize that Haitian people are not like African people! Which means that what works in Africa won't necessarily work in Haiti. Cultural norms in Haiti need to be considered and not put on the same plate with other low-resourced countries, even if they may be African.

Change takes time and energy. One of the things I saw as a source of resistance is the habit that some foreign professionals have of criticizing what we already have: the system is bad, nothing is working, and everything needs to be changed. Haitian nurses are not looking for a savior. They are good at many things. They're in their own country and know their population. They look for people who can guide them in the right direction without forcing or criticizing. Changing a system may seem fascinating, but putting a durable and viable changed system in place by using local nurses and engaging them in a way that embraces your vision—as if it is theirs—is more than amazing.

MY FIRST JOB

My first job was at Hospital Albert Schweitzer (HAS), a private hospital in the community of Deschapelles in the Artibonite Valley in a rural area of Haiti. The hospital was founded in the 1950s by Dr. Larimer Mellon, a member of a wealthy American family who were contemporaries of the Rockefellers. (Paris, 2000) With a capacity of 210 beds in 2003, HAS was a good place to start as a novice nurse. They were using an American system very different and more organized than the one I was familiar with. I was impressed with their medical equipment and supplies—very different from the National Hospital in Port-au-Prince, where I had done my clinical rotations as a student. At the National Hospital patients had to buy everything, which often delayed treatment because of their poor economic situation. At HAS the care was virtually free—a small fee of 48 gdes (~$1.00 U.S.) was paid by the patient and everything was included: consultation, medication, and lab work. At HAS I felt useful as a nurse. Patient care was not delayed because of lack of medication or supplies. I was exposed to good techniques such as resuscitation and participated more often in saving lives than I was able to as a student. It was fantastic! After 1 year of clinical practice I was promoted to nurse manager of the pediatric ward. This wonderful experience helped me develop my leadership and management abilities. In that position nursing care was seen in a different way. It wasn't just about doing a great job, but also about making sure that my team was strong enough to give appropriate and safe care to our patients. In that way, teaching my colleagues was a priority. I started to be a teacher and a preceptor. I used classroom and bedside teaching methods while I continued to improve my clinical competencies.

I have met nurses from the United States, Switzerland, and Canada. They are teachers as well as nurses and very experienced. They taught me a lot about preceptor roles, evidence-based practice, and communication. Through collaboration with them I was able to travel to Switzerland for an intensive 3-month training in neonatology, which enabled me to advance from nurse manager to nurse coordinator at HAS.

ZANMI LASANTE

In 2007, after almost 4 years, I decided to leave HAS to move to the Central Plateau, to work for Zanmi Lasante (ZL). Another great experience was begun!

ZL, a sister program of Partners in Health (PIH), works to improve the quality of health care in the public health system in Haiti. (Kidder, 2003) The goal of ZL is to empower existing local governmental health facilities.

ZL has eleven sites, eight in the Central Plateau and three in the Artibonite. I was assigned to Cange. Things were very different from what I had known at HAS. For the first time I learned about chemotherapy. I was able to apply my new skills with a 3-year-old boy, one of our pediatric patients, who had Wilms' Tumor. Up until then I thought it was over for somebody in Haiti who had cancer. ZL showed me there's still hope. I am writing these words with a smile on my face, because I remember the smile of this boy's father when the pediatrician told him: "Sir, we cannot say we're going to save your son, but we're going to do everything we can to save him. The good news is that the chemo medications are in Port-au-Prince and will be in Cange this evening. The chemotherapy will be started tomorrow." I will never forget this father's smile and the hope and gratitude I could read in his eyes. This little boy's family was very poor and could never have afforded chemo treatment. ZL offered them the treatment without having to pay anything. It's not like I agree with some nongovernmental organizations that increase the dependence of the population by offering them everything and not encouraging them to take their life in their own hands and participate in their care. But I think about the beauty of saving a life others would consider to be over. There are facilities in Haiti where, whatever the illness or the severity of the health problem, without money a patient needs to find another place. Is that a bad thing? Let's look at an example: I went with one of my patients, a 4-year-old boy who had cancer, to a hospital in Port-au-Prince to admit him for one night. This patient had an appointment the next day at the U.S. Embassy for a visa to go to Boston for chemo and radiation therapy. He had ascites and was oxygen dependent. The hospital refused to accept the patient for the insane reason that they didn't want to increase their pediatric mortality rate. I was shocked and had to advocate for him with the medical director of the hospital. I called one of the board members of ZL to help me convince the medical director that the patient was not going to die during the night. In my opinion, not only as a nurse but as a human being, no statistic can be more important than a life.

PATIENT EDUCATION AND ADVOCACY

Patient advocacy is not really part of the education of most of the nurses that I've worked with. The cultural norm is that the medical team exercises complete control over the patient. Acceptance of this approach is observed most in facilities with vulnerable patients who can't pay for medical care. In many situations I have felt as if the medical team is against the patient. What I say may seem like an excessive conclusion; however, let's be concrete. The patient has the right to understand his diagnosis, his medications, and why he has to take them. One method medical teams sometimes use to obtain consent is to scare the patient: "If you don't take the medication or if you don't stay in the hospital or if you don't accept this intervention you're going to die." This statement doesn't necessarily reflect a patient's true condition but is used to achieve compliance. I don't believe the medical team does this with a bad purpose in mind. I suppose they believe they are acting for the good of the patient. However, I learned from an American nurse another way to encourage compliance, and it works—patient education. I had a patient who refused a blood transfusion. His hemoglobin was 6g/dl. He looked very pale and had shortness of breath. Transfusion was necessary. The medical team tried different methods to convince the patient he was going to die if not transfused, which was not totally false in his situation. They tried to threaten the patient: "If you don't want us to help you, why don't you go home?" This American nurse and I chose a different approach. We discussed the situation with the patient—in clear and concise words. He understood the issues at stake and finally accepted the transfusion.

Threatening or scaring patients doesn't work. The role of the medical team (nurses and doctors) is not to decide for the patient but to give clear information to help him make the right decision for himself.

The training we provided for the team in an attempt to change their way of thinking was exhausting but fruitful. Change takes time and energy. One or two days of training isn't enough to reach that goal. It takes constant work and practice.

RESPECT FOR OTHER'S BELIEFS

Working in a poor country like mine—Haiti—is a wonderful experience for foreign health care providers. It gives them the opportunity to think about nursing care and patient safety as well as cultural beliefs and approaches. In Haiti, patients often rely on herbal medicine. Understanding the interaction between a medication and the tea that a patient is taking at the same time is not always obvious. Other beliefs have to do with religion. An HIV patient can stop taking highly active antiretroviral therapy (HAART) because he trusts that God is going to heal him. Another strong cultural belief is "voodoo." Voodoo has its origins in West Africa and combines spirituality with health care practices. (Hoodoo, once practiced in the southern United States, has similar roots.)

A patient's family came to the ward and asked the doctor to discharge their family member because they were sure the patient's problem was not medical but mystical. The 12-year-old boy had peritonitis and had undergone surgical exploration. An American pediatric nurse from Boston, the pediatrician, the surgeon, and I tried in vain to explain to the parents the illness, the procedure, and why it was important for the boy to stay in the hospital—all without success. The father was convinced their neighbor wanted to kill his boy and transform him into a zombie. We knew the boy was going to die if he left the hospital. The team was facing an ethical dilemma. In Haiti, there are no rules or policies to protect patients' rights. In this case we did not have the legal right to stop the parents and keep the child. They left the hospital with the sick boy without medical consent. They went to the Houngan a voodoo priest. Unfortunately, 8 days later his parents brought him back to us and he died 2 hours after admission.

It wasn't the first case, in my experience, where the parents or the patient left the hospital because they believed their condition was not medical. Sometimes I got the chance to convince parents or patients to stay and delay their *Houngan* consultation. Haitian health care providers have to deal with these issues and it's not easy at all.

These are the types of cases where community health agents (ajan de santé) can intervene to prevent regrettable situations. One role of the community health agent is to go into the community to provide education for the *Houngan*. We cannot stop the *Houngan* because many people trust in them. But with respectful education they often become allies and refer their clients to the hospital before their condition becomes too advanced to treat. Our culture is amazing and rich. Nevertheless its complexity can be misunderstood and hurt families. When dealing with these cases I always show respect for their religion even if it's different from mine. I try to recognize the importance that voodoo has for them and show them how medical science can complement their beliefs. This conversation is often tricky and I realize that one wrong word about their faith or the power of their priest and the patient's trust in me will disappear.

NURSING EDUCATION IN HAITI

Before closing, I would like to say something about nursing education. The nursing team is composed of registered nurses (RNs), Auxiliaires (more or less an equivalent to a licensed practical nurse [LPN]), and Patient Care Attendants (PCAs), a new component providing community outreach. Requirements to become an RN depend on the school. A nurse from one of the national schools must complete 3 years of courses and clinical rotations plus 1 year of social service before graduating from the program. The degree earned is a diploma. The RN license is obtained after a national exam, which allows the nurse to work anywhere in the country. The licensing exam is administered by the Ministère de la Santé Publique et de la Population (MSPP), Haiti's Ministry of Health. Haiti has four national schools: one in Port-au-Prince, the capital of Haiti; one in Cayes; one in Cap-Haitian; and the fourth in Jeremie. Those four national schools have essentially the same curriculum. In January 2014, a new curriculum for nursing education submitted by the Direction des Soins Infirmiers (DSI)—Haiti's Board of Nursing—was approved by the Ministry of Health. That means that these nursing programs will change from 3 years to

4 years and will become part of the national university system; a big step for the profession in Haiti.

In addition to the national schools, there are 45 private accredited nursing schools. Some schools have a 4-year program, others 3 years and their curriculum is variable and unknown. Nurses from private schools can apply for the national exam to be licensed. The Auxiliaires complete a 9-month program with a different curriculum from the RN programs. PCAs are people with a minimum education who are from the community. They don't have formal medical or nursing training but are trained by the nursing team in the hospital. The wide variability among these programs can affect nursing work and collaboration.

Continuing education of health care providers has been a challenge in Haiti, where the health care system doesn't always reflect reality and is removed from the technological developments and changes we see around the world. Diseases seen in other places can be very different from what we are used to dealing with.

In a limited-resource country such as Haiti, one of the key factors to ensure quality care is to empower the local work force through support and training. I have been fortunate to receive and provide both.

As I look back on my career, I remember that women who died so long ago and realize that the greatest lesson I have learned is that being part of a medical team and working with vulnerable people requires heart, passion, and compassion. I feel fortunate to work in a setting where I can use these attributes to help improve health in my region of Haiti.

REFERENCES

Kidder, T. (2003). *Mountains beyond mountains: The quest of Dr. Paul Farmer, a man who would cure the world*. New York, NY: Random House.

Paris, B. (2000). *Song of Haiti: The lives of Dr. Larimer and Gwen Mellon at the Albert Schweitzer Hospital of Deschapelles*. New York, NY: Public Affairs.

8

Comparing Health Systems

A Scottish Nurse Finds Herself in North Carolina

LINDA JOSEPH

Editor's Note: The focus of Linda Joseph's chapter is quite different from that of others in this collection. Linda describes her experience moving from the United Kingdom to eventually becoming licensed in the United States. She shares her observations regarding nursing practice in the United States as she compares her experience with the U.S. health care system with that of the United Kingdom. Given debate in the United States regarding access to health care, her comments, as an outsider, are thought-provoking.

I am a school nurse in North Carolina. I have been a nurse for 30 years, although I took a few years off to have my children. I have three children who are now in their twenties and a husband with whom I have been married for nearly 30 years. My husband works for a global biotech company and my sons have now graduated with their bachelor's degrees; my oldest son also has his masters in medical physics. My younger son is a certified athletic trainer and is now applying to graduate schools, and my daughter is in pharmacy school, and she will graduate in 2017 with her PharmD. All will have careers in health.

I attended high school in Motherwell, Scotland, where I remember my interview with the career advisor. As soon as I mentioned I was interested in nursing, she asked if I knew how to apply and then the interview came to an abrupt end—I guess I was one of the easy ones! I cannot actually remember how or why I decided on nursing—it was so long ago. I was 17 years old then. I started nursing school in Glasgow, Scotland, where after graduating I worked in a peripheral vascular surgery unit at the Glasgow Royal Infirmary. Glasgow Royal Infirmary was built in the 18th and 19th centuries. Although additions have been added throughout the 20th century, I remember the traditional "nightingale" wards with their polished wooden floors and Nursing Officers (Matrons) who were formal and strict. It was steeped in tradition with a bust of James Lister, who developed the practice of antisepsis—in the main entrance.

I married and moved 400 miles to Reading, England. Even this relatively small move took some adjustments. I worked in a much smaller hospital, which was a big change from the university teaching hospital I had come from. After about a year I moved to a larger hospital that was also nearer home and where I was able to develop my career. A few years later, I was promoted to "Ward Sister." I am not sure that term is used in the United States, but another name could be Charge Nurse or Ward Manager. It was a busy surgical Urology ward, with 30 beds and about 15 nurses. Looking back, this is where I became interested in patient health education and supporting nursing students. I was particularly interested in the care of patients with testicular cancer, and as part of a short course at the University of Reading I was able to research the disease and spent a week visiting the most famous cancer hospital in the country, the Royal Marsden Hospital in London. I enjoyed my position for about 2 years until I became pregnant with my first child, and after my maternity leave I decided to become a full-time mum (or mom, as you say in the United States).

PUBLIC OR PRIVATE HEALTH CARE

All of my nursing until this point had taken place in National Health Service (NHS) hospitals. The NHS provides free national health care (no copays) for everyone in the United Kingdom. This is provided by the government, paid for by taxes under the management of local health authorities. There are some horror stories about people having to wait for treatment, however these are generally isolated examples and I believe the NHS generally does a great job providing health care for the UK population. There are often waiting lists for nonurgent surgery, but in serious illnesses where time is critical the NHS does well. Recently, I have had personal experience with the NHS because my dad, who still lives in Scotland, has required several operations in the last 5 years; partial colectomy, triple artery bypass, and a knee replacement. On all of these occasions, I have been really impressed with the care he received in the hospital and the follow-up care in the community. All of his care was covered by the NHS and prescriptions in Scotland are also free for retired citizens. My U.S. friends and colleagues often ask me about our health care system and seem amazed that I have positive comments.

While my children were small, I worked part time as a registered nurse (RN) in a private hospital. This was a very different experience for me; this hospital was more like a hotel than a hospital. They mainly provided planned surgery for people who had private health insurance as an employment benefit; this enabled them to choose when the surgery should take place to suit their work and family needs. This hospital did a variety of surgical procedures and surgeries but had no intensive care unit or emergency department, emergency care required transfer to the local NHS hospital. Senior doctors and surgeons usually worked under contract with the NHS, but also had a private practice which supplemented their income. Private health insurance companies were then billed for the treatments. This was an interesting experience but not as rewarding as the NHS positions I had held. While there, I applied for and was successful in getting my first school nurse position.

MORE THAN A "NIT NURSE"

As a school nurse in Berkshire, I covered five schools, the equivalent of K–12. I was an NHS employee and our team of nurses was based in a local community health center, spending on average 1 day per week in a school. Due to the limited time in individual schools, most of our time was spent training school staff and student screening; vision/hearing/height/weight. The demographic of the school population was mixed, from very wealthy families to families who relied on social security allowances. There was really no immigrant population at that time, so language was not a barrier to communication with students or parents. However, I believe that this has changed as more families move to the United Kingdom from Eastern Europe.

One of my responsibilities was to staff a weekly sexual health clinic at the high school with the highest teenage pregnancy rate. The team consisted of a school nurse, a doctor, and a youth worker.

Contraception advice and prescription information were provided as well as testing for sexually transmissible infections, counseling, and referrals. In preparation for this role, I completed a university course in contraception and sexual health, thereby broadening my development as a public health nurse with an interest in sexual health.

MOVING TO THE UNITED STATES

I really did not choose to work as a nurse internationally. Just as everything seemed settled, my husband was offered a 3-year assignment with his company at their offices in North Carolina. It was a great offer, and moving from the United Kingdom to the United States did not seem so daunting because we knew we had the option to return home. All of our family still lived in Scotland. They were surprised but supportive of our decision, and had visited us numerous times. So after two visits to North Carolina and successful visa applications, we packed our container and our family of five plus two cats and moved to Chapel Hill, NC.

One of our first priorities was to settle our children into school. I found the schools to be very welcoming and helpful toward them. Interestingly, one of the biggest challenges for my children was learning the measuring system, as UK schools had been teaching the metric system since the 1970s. I had to tackle the task of setting up doctors and dentists, negotiate which provider we could visit, what in and out of network meant, copays, and the amount not covered by insurance. All of this is a huge learning curve when your normal is to just sign up at a doctor's office nearby and not worry about how it is paid for. We needed tax ID numbers to get our driver licenses. Only my husband was allowed a social security number. We had to learn to drive on the other side of the road and how to negotiate a 4-way stop!

My first contact with school nursing in North Carolina was when I got a letter from the school nurse advising me that my daughter's immunizations were incomplete. I had 30 days to get her DTaP or she would be suspended from school. Immunizations are not required in the United Kingdom, but most parents do voluntarily immunize their children. I called the nurse to say that my daughter had been given her 4th shot. I was told it would have to be repeated because it had been given before her 4th birthday. When I asked "why" I expected a research-based answer, but was simply told because it is North Carolina law. I always remember this experience when I approach new families about immunization records.

Moving from one country to another is a challenge. Visas are complicated. The type of visa I had did not permit me to work, so I went back to school and completed my BS in Public Health. This was a great opportunity that allowed me to study many areas of interest, such as teenage pregnancy and testicular cancer. I was able to develop a testicular self-exam leaflet. My final paper dealt with childhood obesity, which continues to be a priority for school nursing.

During this time, we traveled within the United States, trying to see as much as possible. The highlights include Yosemite National Park and the Grand Canyon. We were also able to make yearly visits back to the UK where our family was quick to point out the change in our children's accents. However, most of our Scottish family and friends thought the new American accents were preferable to the original English accents—Scotland and England have a lot of history!

"GREEN CARDS"

Toward the end of his work contract, my husband was offered a permanent position in the United States. We decided to stay. It really wasn't a difficult decision. We felt settled and our children were doing well in school. However, in order to remain "legal," we had to leave the country to renew our visas, so we made a weekend trip to Calgary, Canada in the middle of winter (extremely cold!). The trip was not like a vacation at all. It was quite a surreal experience. We left home with the knowledge that if our visas were not renewed we could not return! We visited the American Consulate and waited. Our applications were taken and we were told to return in 2 days to collect our passports and visas. Fortunately, everything was in order and we returned home. Shortly afterward we started the "green card," or permanent resident, applications. This is a long process of applications and medicals. We all needed chest x-rays to check for tuberculosis, as we had received the Bacillus Calmette–Guérin (BCG) vaccine in the United Kingdom and would therefore have a positive skin test. We all made several trips to Charlotte for fingerprinting and photographs. My daughter was called back for another appointment. Letters from the Immigration and Naturalization Service (INS) never give any details or explanations and—even when you get there—immigration officers really don't explain very much at all. Each building has security similar to an airport, where all bags have to be x-rayed. We all eventually received our green cards but not all at the same time. Once I had my green card I felt more secure living in the United States and I was able to apply for a job.

BACK TO WORK!

With my degree in public health, I found a position as a health educator at the Poe Center for Health Education in Raleigh. They provide health education for K–12 students in a purpose-built center or by traveling to schools within North Carolina. The center has several themed lecture theaters; body systems, dental, drugs, nutrition, and family life. It was a great experience. My work involved family life education where—before starting work—I was advised about what questions I could and could not answer. The experience offered an opportunity to develop presentation skills to keep kids interested and involved. I also learned new computer skills and assisted with updating and developing programs. In addition to the educational activities offered at the Poe Center, we also developed programs for the schools. I visited many schools and presented classes—primarily in sexual health—to 5th, 7th, and 9th/10th graders. I hope that the children benefited from the classes offered by the Poe Center.

BECOMING LICENSED

I missed being a nurse and the continuity of care that comes with getting to know those under your care. I felt I needed to do more than health education. So I started the process of becoming an RN in the United States. Fortunately, I had maintained my nursing registration in the United Kingdom, as this was a requirement to apply in the United States. After some research, I found that the North Carolina Board of Nursing (NCBON) requires international nurses to be approved by the Commission on Graduates of Foreign Nursing Schools (CGFNS), so I started the process. They offer two routes. One is the CGFNS exam, which is usually the option for newly qualified nurses who plan to work in the United States. I remember these exams were held in large hotels in the United Kingdom, for nurses who were planning to move to the United States. They also offer a credential evaluation route, which provides a detailed analysis of the credentials earned at multiple levels of nursing education from outside the United States according to what is required for individual states. I chose this option. Not only did it avoid an exam, but it provided an evaluation of all of my continuing education since I had become an RN, including my degree in public health, and is therefore the best option for nurses who are not newly registered. The process involved completing applications and the huge task of gathering transcripts from my high school, nursing school, and university. Some of this was extremely challenging as it had been more than 20 years since I had qualified as an RN. After several months I received a report from the CGFNS, which recognized that my qualifications were equivalent to U.S. nursing qualifications. The North Carolina Board of Nursing (NCBON) also required international nurses to take an English proficiency exam, but as I am from the United Kingdom I was exempt! With all of this completed, I was allowed to apply to take the National Council Licensure Examination (NCLEX).

I started studying for the NCLEX. It was a huge challenge for me, not only because it had been a long time since I completed nursing school, but multiple choice testing was completely alien to me. In the United Kingdom most exams in high schools and universities are essay questions, and coursework and dissertations are a considerable part of a student's grade. I was a 40-something year old trying to study for a new style of exam. I bought all the study guides and buried myself in test questions.

It had been a long time since nursing school, medicine had moved forward, and all of the abbreviations and spelling in the United Kingdom and United States are so different! Even blood sugar and cholesterol levels are measured on different scales. For all of these reasons the NCLEX was a huge challenge for me and at times I asked myself why I was putting myself through this agony. I eventually passed and once again could call myself a nurse!

A few weeks before the exam date, I saw a school nurse position advertised at a local high school. I had previously met the coordinator of Health/Student Services when she attended one of my Poe Center presentations, so I called her to discuss the vacancy. She encouraged me to apply and the interview went well, but the principal did not want to wait for me to get my "ducks in a row" and the position was offered to another nurse. Once my "ducks got in a row" I started the search for a job. The school year was just about to start but there seemed to be nothing available in the school districts nearby. I really didn't want to return to working unsociable hours and weekends, so I started looking at hospital clinic positions. I had several interviews and was offered a position.

However, at the same time, I was contacted by the nurse manager who had interviewed me while I was waiting to take the exam. She told me about a school nurse position in a neighboring district and recommended me to that manager. Within a week I had interviewed and gotten the job! I am so grateful to her for her support and belief in me.

Although I had been in and around schools since my move from the United Kingdom, joining the school staff brought a steep learning curve, and I am thankful for the support of my colleagues. I have now been a school nurse in the United States for 6 years; I am employed by the school system and based in a middle school, but am also responsible for the alternative school in the district. We are extremely lucky in our county to have a school nurse in each school. It allows me to get to know my students and allows me to care for them on a much higher level. The school population is rural with pockets of wealthier districts and has a high Hispanic population—I wish I had learned to speak Spanish. I think I was a novelty to the staff and students when I first joined the school. Even now, when a new staff member is hired or the new 6th grade arrives, my accent is a great form of entertainment. Some teachers joke that students come to see me not because they are ill but just to hear me speak! Whatever the reason, I feel I add to their global awareness by simply being there. We often have conversations about the United Kingdom or immigration to the United States. I believe nursing is a profession that lends itself to global transitions. It may be easier for nurses to make the transition because being a nurse requires you to be caring, to collaborate well with colleagues, and to be a good communicator with colleagues and those you care for. I would definitely encourage other nurses to consider working abroad. Although my experience is limited to the United Kingdom and the United States, it has been extremely valuable to see different ways of doing things and to learn to adapt.

When I was first asked to participate in this book, I was confused as I had not really considered myself to be a "global nurse"; the United States and United Kingdom are similar in many ways, but there are lots of differences too. With the Hispanic population growing, there are many cultural and language barriers to overcome within the United States. Dealing with immunization compliance is complicated by foreign immunization records; children are often missing required vaccines or have had dosages outside the recommendations. We have some interpreters within the school district, but there is a definite need for more. We have English as a Second Language (ESL) program in the schools, but often children have little or no English when they start school. It is amazing to see how quickly they learn. It is often much harder for their parents—particularly their mothers—which can make it difficult to communicate regarding their children's health needs.

THE PATH TO CITIZENSHIP

Immigration is a long process; when you have held your green card for 5 years you become eligible to apply for citizenship. There are more applications to complete and fees to pay; at the time we applied it cost about $600 each. After the applications were submitted, I studied for the English and Civics test that had to be taken at the required interview. There is a study book of 100 questions. You are asked 10 questions at your interview and must answer 6 correctly. I remember a Jay Leno show where he asked these questions of Americans and they didn't get very many correct! After successfully completing the interview process, we were given a date to attend the Naturalization Ceremony where my family became U.S. citizens. During the ceremony the immigration officer declared, "You are now free of U.S. immigration!" This line got a laugh from almost everyone in the room. Our green cards were taken away and we were given a certificate of naturalism. I must admit this certificate did not seem strong enough to prove our citizenship, so very quickly we applied for U.S. passports. It was a good feeling to finally become a citizen. We felt more secure living here—free of the worry that we could have our green card revoked and be asked to leave the country. Also, we finally had the right to vote; for years we had been experiencing "taxation without representation."

NATIONAL CERTIFICATION AS A SCHOOL NURSE

My testing was not yet over. My current school nurse position requires us to become a Nationally Certified School Nurse within 3 years of the start of employment. So I began studying for another test and in 2010 I added this qualification to my playbook.

In my current position I enjoy caring for the busy day-to-day needs of my school population. My colleagues are supportive and help when I am "lost in translation." I have extra responsibilities within my role, I am currently the chairperson of the county's School Health Advisory Council (SHAC), I am a preceptor for student nurses who are completing their public health module, and I am the nurse coordinator for student health education.

In comparison to my school nurse position in the United Kingdom, my current job is much more fulfilling; I not only deal with illness and injuries for students and staff, but also screening and assessment of children with health concerns. I am also involved with student support services, working closely with our school social worker and school counselors to help students achieve success and assess/refer any mental health concerns. This includes being involved with the assessment of students who have suicidal thoughts or ideas. It is concerning how often this occurs, and I am reassured by the policies and protocols we have in our school district to help guide us.

I still wear my health educator "hat." I train staff to be proficient in first aid/CPR, medication administration, and diabetes care. My involvement with sexual/reproductive health and education has also continued. I recently participated in the transition to a new health curriculum within our district's middle and high schools. We moved to comprehensive sexual health education and away from the abstinence-only education that was previously in place—to ensure our school district is in compliance with the North Carolina Healthy Youth Act 2009. With implementation of the Healthy Youth Act students have more information with which to make informed choices. However, there is still more to do. Based on my experience in the United Kingdom nearly 10 years ago, it seems the United Kingdom is ahead of the United States in regards to sexual health education for children. Parents in the United Kingdom seemed more open to "sex ed" and understood the need for the school-based clinic I discussed earlier. I am not sure that North Carolina parents are ready for that!

In the United Kingdom our team of nurses saw each other at the beginning and end of each day. It was a useful time to discuss concerns and get support from other professional nurses. In the United States I feel more like a sole practitioner. I always remind my student nurses that working in a school environment is very different from working in a hospital, where backup is always available or where you can get another professional opinion when you need it. Our nursing team has monthly meetings and we each provide backup to another school nurse. We have our own additional responsibilities and have subgroups that work to keep our resources updated. My colleagues are a great group of nurses with a wide range of experience. Listening to them helps me to acclimatize to American health jargon. I share some British health information. Recently they all enjoyed the British Heart Foundation's video promoting hands-only cardiopulmonary resuscitation (CPR), which features actor Vinnie Jones and Stayin' Alive by the Bee Gees. Sometimes I completely confuse them; recently I mentioned a friend who was a theater nurse. They all assumed she was a nurse who worked in a theater! In the United Kingdom we call our operating rooms "operating theaters!"

THOUGHTS FOR THE FUTURE

My family and I have had good experiences with health care in the United States. Sometimes I think providers do more testing, more frequently than needed, when more could be assessed from the health history. However, in general we have been well cared for through our employee health insurance plans. In contrast, for some of my students I am their only health care. This is one of my main concerns about health care in the United States. Many of my students do not have insurance. Their parents often tell their children to see me if they have had a concern the previous day or over the weekend. When I conduct vision screens for students who do not have insurance—and they fail and are referred for further testing—I help families get vision tests and glasses through charitable organizations. I often have students on medication for mental health reasons or attention deficit hyperactivity disorder (ADHD). Sometimes they run out of medication and cannot afford any more for periods of time. Sometimes even students who have insurance use up their allowance for mental health and their therapy ends. I find parents who have insurance are often reluctant to take their child to the doctor or emergency room as they worry about the cost of the copay. These problems are hard to understand since I come from the United Kingdom where our National Health Service (NHS) has been in place for nearly 100 years. It will be interesting to follow the roll-out of the Affordable Care Act here in the United States, in hopes that it will alleviate some of my students' problems.

9

Missionary Nursing

Life Among an Indonesian Tribe

TREVOR C. JOHNSON
TERESA JOHNSON

Editor's Note: Trevor Johnson and his wife Teresa write with humor and insight about their choice to live and work among a very remote tribe in Indonesia. They provide compelling examples regarding differences in world view and how they strive to understand and respect those differences. They also comment on their children's lives as they raise a family under what seems, to Western eyes, to be very difficult circumstances. Interestingly, a look back at Marie Donahue's Chapter 1 offers insight into one of their vignettes.

> If anyone has material possessions and sees his brother in need but has no pity on him, how can the love of God be in him? Dear children, let us not love with words or tongue but with actions and in truth.
>
> –1 John 3:17-18

My wife and I are missionary nurses living among a remote tribal group in the jungles of Indonesia. We use the local language and live among the local people in an attempt to serve them holistically in any way that we can. While we feel that we have already adjusted and

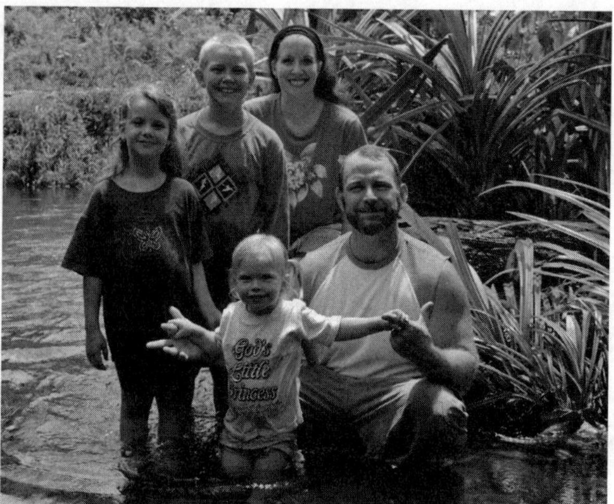

Figure 9.1 The family of Trevor and Teresa Johnson in their bathing spot in Danowage, with children Noah (9), and his two little sisters, Alethea (7) and Perpetua (2).

adapted much (and are still adjusting and adapting), we now have a much healthier respect for the huge role that culture and worldview play in every person's life. People strain, and can even break, when trying to cross cultures. We ourselves felt that strain. Culture and worldview impacts every major decision of life, even how we filter and interpret the world around us. We are unaware of it mostly, and yet, it envelopes us like water around a fish.

We know the stresses of nursing and ministering to others in a culture not our own. Yet, we also know the deep joys of enlarging one's view of the world. We are now enabled to better see this truth: the whole human race is but one solitary quilt or fabric, though woven with many different types and colors of thread, and the world is a much more beautiful place because of it.

OUR PREPARATION

We are both graduates of Deaconess College of Nursing's BSN program (now Chamberlain College of Nursing), in St. Louis, Missouri. An Army Reserve Officers' Training Corps (ROTC) scholarship through Washington University paid my college education in full in exchange for active duty time spent in the army.

I chose nursing in order to serve God by serving others. The Catholic Saint Teresa of Avila once stated that Jesus has no body on earth now but ours, "*. . . Yours are the feet with which he walks to do good. Yours are the hands through which he blesses all the world . . .*" I desired to follow such a calling, to be the hands and feet of Jesus in some small way, particularly to those living remotely and without access to other medical help.

This sense of calling was confirmed during a short-term trip to the remote Amazon River. There, I delivered a baby on the floor of a dirty hut along the banks of that gargantuan water. Lacking proper supplies, I tied off the cord with a hammock string boiled over an earthen clay hearth and cut the cord with a Wilkerson shaving razor. Dogs underneath the house peered between rough-hewn floorboards and lapped up the drippings. We used our drinking water for the infant's first bath. Returning home via small metal canoe (a mere speck on that wide expanse of water), we wilted under the searing sun until we stopped at a village to seek refreshment. My thirst was quenched by a strange frothy, orange cassava drink. I queasily learned later that women sat around such vats, spitting into these concoctions in order to ferment the mixture into a form of local beer. Yuck!

Two days later in another village, a man with a gray and sweaty pallor rasped out a plea for help. He was suffering chest tightness and clutched at his left shoulder with numb fingers. I was able to give him donated nitroglycerin tablets. Within minutes his color returned and his breathing stabilized. This greatly impacted me. This truth dawned on me: In America I could get a decent job with a good wage. Every major town has a clinic or hospital. In remote regions like this, on the other hand, I might very well be the difference between life and death. I pondered, *"If ten men are hoisting a heavy uneven log, and nine of them are heaving on the little end and only one is laboring to hold up the heavy end—and I want to help, which end should I lift?"* I resolved then and there to find the most remote peoples left on earth and to seek to serve them.

I gained not only a solid degree from nursing school, but I also gained a wonderful wife. Teresa was not only smart and well-trained, but was pretty as a doll in her nursing uniform. What a perfectly suited partner she makes now as we labor together in an unhealthy jungle region and treat the sick. How my heart is pulled as I see her unselfish compassion toward others. To watch her play with our children is as close to heaven on earth as one can get. Our home is very well-lived in. It is raucous, and messy, littered with battalions of army men and ruined remains of Lego cities. Child art taped at all angles adorns every wall (mostly unicorns or army men . . . and, at least once, army men riding unicorns). I wouldn't have it any other way.

I served 5 years active duty as an army officer in the Army Nurse Corps, a great place to gain experience in those first few years of nursing. The army provided some very helpful training for our future in the jungle, such as the Tactical Care of the Combat Casualty (TCCC) course and also some training such as Advanced Cardiac Life Support (ACLS) which, while much appreciated during my time working in a hospital, has not proved very useful in this low-technology environment. Machine-dependent nursing practices have largely given way to community health preventative measures (don't poop where you drink, boil your water, and bathe regularly) as well as a "ditch medicine" mentality here due to our locale. Teresa worked as a community health nurse at Fort Leonard Wood, Missouri, focusing on immunizations and communicable disease tracking and prevention. Her background has proven most useful in tribal work.

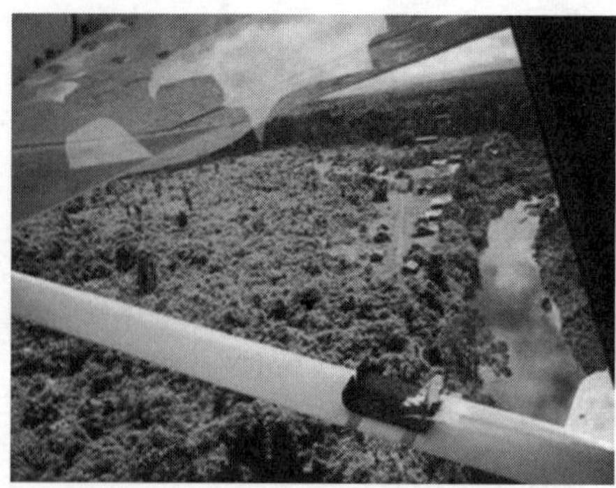

Figure 9.2 Final approach by MAF (Missionary Aviation Fellowship) floatplane onto our river strip, Swampy International Airport. Danowage village on the left bank.

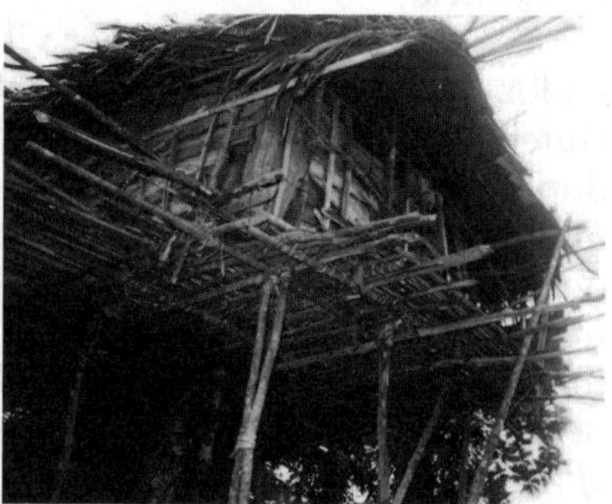

Figure 9.3 Typical Korowai treehouse.

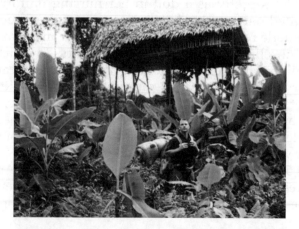

Figure 9.4 Trekking post to post with medicine.

A SNAPSHOT OF OUR LOCATION

National Geographic calls the inhabitants of our region "The Treehouse People," 4,000 semi-nomadic tribal souls. These tribal people live spread out over several hundred kilometers of dense lowland jungle in southern Papua, on the eastern end of the nation of Indonesia. The Mission Aviation Fellowship pilot who lands here calls our area "the most remote area in an already remote land" and "about the furthest place from anywhere." On "plane day" his floatplane sets down with a splash on our narrow river (a river that is often not landable due to wide fluctuations in depth, making medical evacuations dicey during dry season). There are no roads, no electricity, and no land airstrips yet in this broad region. Governmental presence is only now being felt. Two years ago, this tribe was counted in the Indonesian census for the first time.

Two dozen villages and many treehouse clusters dot this vast green expanse. Two dialects of about 2,000 speakers each divide this area roughly in half between north and south. A Dutch translator labors in the southern dialect of the Korowai and is making linguistic progress. We live in the centrally located village of Danowage further upriver among the northern dialect (*The Korowai Batu*, or Rock Korowai) and are partnering with 17 indigenous Christians from the highland Dani tribe trying to improve the lives of those living throughout this broad region.

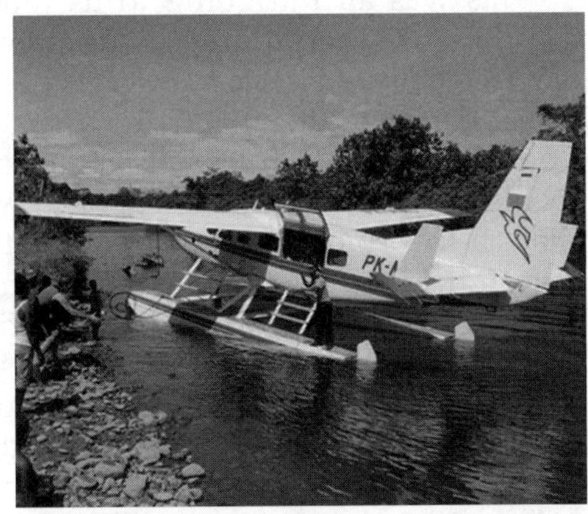

Figure 9.5 Tying up the airplane at our "harbor" in Danowage to unload supplies.

SURPRISES UPON REACHING THE ISLAND OF JAVA

Let's back up a step or two, however, before we land in the jungle. Our first stop in Indonesia was on the island of Java, where we first learned the national language of Indonesian (and yes, they do, in fact, have great coffee in Java). The city of Bandung in West Java possesses many of the amenities of a modern city (they even have a McDonald's). Despite Java being a great place to "land softly" before moving more remotely, it was there that we first became deeply aware of just how much culture and worldview impacts all aspects of life, including health care. Below are some examples:

"*Masuk Angin*" (Entering Air)

When we first arrived in West Java, we were baffled. The climate was very hot, yet lots of motorcycle riders wore thick leather jackets (and some even wore them backwards—across the front). Aren't these people burning up in this tropical heat? Why would they do this? The answer was, "To prevent *masuk angin* (entering air)."

What?!

Yes, many Indonesians believe that air rushing into your body can cause flu-like symptoms. The solution is to apply rubbing oil and scrape your skin with a coin (dermabrasion) to release this trapped air. If you prefer round, raised whelps as opposed to red stripes down your back you can always apply "Chinese cupping" to your skin, instead, to draw out this trapped air.

This was all intriguing to us those first "honeymoon" months in Indonesia. Then it grew infuriating. Many of the nearby hospital staff also believed in *masuk angin*. Feelings of cultural superiority rose in us. We fought against many arrogant and ethnocentric thoughts. We reminded ourselves that just a century or two ago in the West, people complained of "the vapors," which was a similar belief. This miasma theory of disease stating that diseases were spread by noxious air held sway for a long time in the West, in contrast to the much more recent germ theory of disease. The dreaded disease of "malaria" (which I have had 14 times now and is responsible for so many tribal deaths here in Papua) even gets its name from the Latin for "bad air." Remember, Florence Nightingale held to this miasma theory of disease! It led her to implement the beneficial practice of maintaining well-ventilated and clean-smelling hospital wards.

These historical excursions into our own mistaken health notions aside, let me ask you: What would you think if you worked with an Indonesian nurse who believed wholeheartedly in "*masuk angin?*" What would you think of your Indonesian nursing counterparts if you discovered red welts on their shoulders from this "*kerok*" coin-rubbing therapy?

Hygiene and Cleanliness Differences

Imagine our surprise when we witnessed used disposable latex gloves being washed with rubbing alcohol and hung out to dry on a clothesline behind the first Indonesian hospital we toured! Trash, including some medical waste, littered the corridors. Then there was that huge rat that greeted me in the hallway.

Littering is a huge problem throughout all of Indonesia. We tried to convince ourselves that this was not a cultural thing, but merely due to inequality of wealth and lack of funding. Many traditional societies are accustomed to wrapping their food in banana leaves and then throwing those leaves aside after use to biodegrade naturally. Some readjustment is required when mass importation of plastic arrives into such a culture. Also, when government infrastructure is limited and those limited services fail to arrange timely pick-up and disposal, garbage tends to accumulate (even when the average Indonesian family produces far less garbage on any given month than the small mountain produced by even the poorest Americans).

Pregnancy Beliefs

We thought we were adjusting pretty well to Indonesian culture after 3 months. Then we got pregnant! With pregnancy came a whole slew of new cultural challenges. Have you ever been asked to drink a glass of water after religious teachers recited special prayers over it? Have you ever been told to wear a pair of miniature scissors at night around your neck to ward off evil spirits? Have you ever been under cultural pressure to bathe in the waters of seven wells, and change your clothes seven times on your seventh month of pregnancy, even passing a live eel down your shirt to ensure a slippery and eel-like (smooth) delivery? Have you ever considered burying your placenta under your windowsill after offering ritual prayers to it and calling it by the name, "sister placenta?"

Cross-Cultural Communication and the Relational "Yes"

Cross-cultural communication also proved a challenge. Language-learning gaffes are always embarrassing. I once called the "village head" (*kepala desa*) the "village coconut" (*kelapa desa*). I once told of Jesus riding a soybean into Jerusalem instead of a donkey (*kedelai* versus *keledai*). I once told a group of men that men ought to make love to their wives publicly, but my intention was merely to express that husband and wife should be able to hold hands in public and show some public affection. I once stated that I desired a "bad wife" (*istri jahat*) instead of a momentary rest (*istirahat*). At least I didn't become an accidental heretic by teaching that Jesus was a *hewan* (a domesticated animal) during Sunday School instead of merely being *heran* (surprised). I once heard of a visiting American speaker opening his overseas speech with the words, "It tickles me to death to be here," only to have this translated by the bewildered interpreter as, "The speaker says to scratch him until he dies!"

Even when we learned Indonesian words, we still had to learn Indonesian patterns of communication. Cross-cultural communication is more than Google-translating replacement words; it means replacing your thought patterns and ways of expression as well. As much as possible, you must enter into the host culture's way of thinking. For example, change the active voice to the passive voice lest you sound rude and accusatory (even if this means that many cars seem to crash themselves and many cups drop themselves). Adopt local idioms, even if this means that a person harboring a hidden agenda has "a shrimp behind the rock."

Words do more than convey information. Cross-cultural communication is also about knowing how people use language relationally. The "relational yes" is one such example. People were always so helpful when I asked for directions in some parts of Java. Yet those directions often sent me even more awry and got me even more lost. Many Indonesians will give you a nice, affirming "relational yes" no matter the reality of a situation. They do not want to tell you "no" or fail to help you. This can be particularly frustrating when conducting health interviews or seeking medical compliance to given health instructions.

CONFRONTING PREJUDICE

At some point in adapting cross-culturally, you will find yourself growing judgmental when encountering different cultural values from your own. Your ethnocentrism will multiply ten-fold. Your prejudices will lie quietly hidden under a veneer of open-mindedness during good times, but will wait for just the right frustrating cultural moment to mutiny and hijack your best thoughts concerning your host culture during your not-so-good times. You will exult one moment in the cultural progress you have gained, and the next moment you will curse "the stupid ways of the locals" under your breathe. Theoretically you will long to love all of mankind, but the rub comes in loving those individual persons you encounter on a day-to-day basis. It seems an unfortunate aspect of human nature that we excuse faults committed by members of our own race, tribe, or in-group and justify them as mere isolated examples (one "bad egg" among an otherwise good group). Faults committed by members of another race, tribe, or culture that are not our own in-group, however, often get attributed to the entire group as a whole. A White person might steal, but Blacks are thieves. A Westerner might tell a lie, but Javanese are liars. It is an ugly feeling, and shameful. For this reason, many Westerners will claim not to harbor such distasteful attitudes. But just immerse yourself in another culture for an extended period of time. Just let yourself experience yet another traffic jam in Jakarta, another pick-pocketing attempt, or another episode of smoking at right-up-in-your face-proximity on public transportation. Many prejudices are far from rational, and many people lack the self-awareness to even realize that they, too, hold such ethnocentric beliefs. The lens by which we see the world is so often smudged. The filter by which we process the raw data of reality is so often marred. We process reality with an empirical bias that gathers alleged "evidences" against our host culture when we grow frustrated with them. Instead of seeing their cultural diversity as a wonderful reflection of God's creativity, worthy of dignity and respect, we become quicker to judge than we are to understand. This happens especially in moments of stress.

Here are two examples. First, I grew up in the Midwest among a farming community where it was a matter of pride to work hard and have calloused hands to show for it. Many upper-class store owners in Java, however, exhibit well-manicured abnormally long thumbnails as a status symbol. Why? It shows that they do not have to engage in manual labor. Every time I see these men, judgment wells up in my breast. Second, I still fight the feeling that many Javanese men appear very creepy toward my

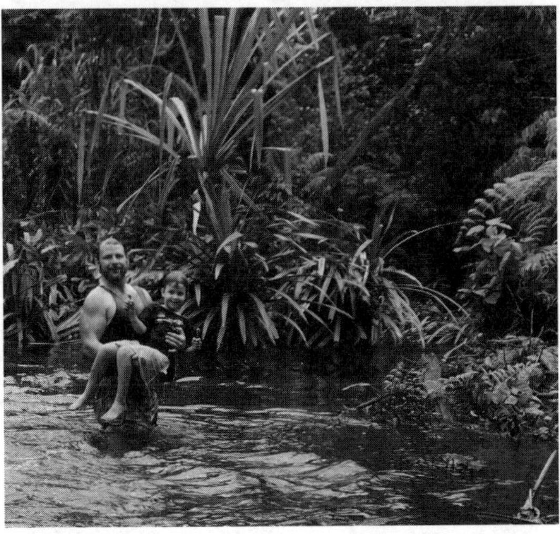

Figure 9.6 Trevor Johnson and daughter Alethea in the family swimming hole, Danowage.

children. They like to pay compliments to my small children, especially my little girls. A matronly Javanese woman telling me about the cuteness of my 6-year-old daughter's dress is endearing. A middle-aged chain-smoking Javanese man calling my daughter pretty, on the other hand, just gives me the willies—even if he is just trying to be nice.

LIVING AMONG A TRIBE

After learning the language in Java for a year, we moved to eastern Indonesia, to the region of West Papua. There we built a house in a jungle village and settled in to live with a tribal group. We now live hundreds of kilometers away from advanced health care. We operate a primitive "health clinic" on our front veranda, our kids beating on a cooking pot to signify its start each afternoon. The walking sick climb our porch to have their symptoms checked. More serious cases involve me trekking out to their huts with meds stowed away in my rucksack.

Living here can be very isolating. As parents of three small children, we are their only health care providers. This can be anxiety-provoking at times of high tropical fever or other injury. As I write this, my daughter lies on a lawn chair, curled up in gastric distress with what seems to be amoeba (again). At least the lone barber in a town only suffers from bad haircuts. What a motivation to stay on top of your craft. However, most tropical illnesses are very predictable and treatable.

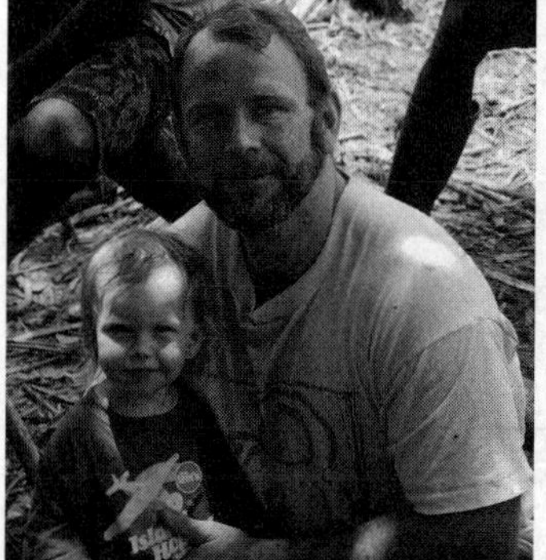

Figure 9.7 Trevor Johnson and daughter Perpetua at a local pig feast.

What about the overall quality of our family life? Are my children deprived? Not at all! Their experiences are richer. They have three rivers to choose from; their usual dilemma is, "Where do I swim now?" They play soccer, climb trees, and hunt bugs (collecting more than I would like to see). They shoot bows and arrows, attend school at home, get dirty, and then visit the river again (wash, rinse, and repeat). They fall into bed at night, usually exhausted from having fun. Rather than entitlement and ingratitude, a sense of thankfulness and awareness of being blessed develops. They see how the less fortunate live. They help me treat the sick. They see both the good and evil of multiple cultures and can weigh and question these worldviews. There is added risk, yes, but all lives are fragile, all plans uncertain, and no place in this broken world is truly safe.

TRIBAL NURSING STORIES

The following are several stories from the past several years that may better illustrate the challenges of missionary nursing among a remote tribe.

"You Raised the Dead!"

Many tribal peoples here assume that the unconscious or unresponsive sick are already dead. It is certainly hard, after all, to verify shallow breathing while in a creaking hut bursting with family members and piglets and without any equipment such as a stethoscope. Upon climbing into the crowded home, I am greeted with the words *"emilo"* and *"sudah mati"* ("already dead" in two languages). I can count at least four clear cases now of rousing such slumbering cases with an injection, infusion, or even simply by wetting their lips with a moist towel or sugar.

"Did He Just Murder His Kid on My Living Room Floor?"

One such sick boy that was prematurely pronounced dead ended up finally dying, most likely by his own father's hands. His shallow breathing was barely perceptible. Further treatment was resisted by his parents. They had already lost hope, and yet there was a pulse. They wanted to bury him immediately and return to their treehouse. When we tried to convince the parents to move the child into our home for closer (and quieter) monitoring, the father was livid, "He's already dead, bury him, we need to get back to our treehouse!" The child improved after IV infusion, his pulse strengthened, and his breathing became perceptible. He had gone without eating or drinking for 3 days, however, and was very weak. The father grew almost violent in his insistence that the child had no hope. He seethed. We gave food to the parents to pacify them, and then put our own kids to bed. They had uneasy questions about our new houseguests, but having critical patients overnight with us has become the norm. We stayed awake and checked on the child often. He had begun swallowing and moving his mouth on his own in response to spoonfuls of juice.

About midnight in our living room, Teresa came upon the father hunched over the child's still warm body. He appeared to have his hands over the child's mouth. The child was no longer breathing. It seemed very suspicious. "He's already dead, let's go," he told his wife, and then told Teresa, "I told you he was going to die." The man then demanded a flashlight from us and stormed out of the house. In the early morning they left the corpse to be buried by our Dani tribal coworkers and trekked home alone. The father was so convinced that the child would die, and so impatient to get home, we believe that the father helped the child to stop breathing.

"Oh No, the Government Health Care Workers Are Coming!"

Many plans to help the poor are ill-conceived, and executed even worse. Two years ago, the Korowai people were "discovered" by the government and listed on the national census for the first time ever, the government census party trekking over 2 weeks to reach our area (I guess they didn't know about our water-strip). Since that time, the government has occasionally sent health care workers upriver to us with mixed results. While we appreciate the fact that we can sometimes receive free medicine, some other practices are alarming. They mass distribute medicine to tribal people who have no understanding of how to store or keep these meds. I have climbed into jungle treehouses only to find white, chalky heaps in the corner—rotting meds! I have seen small children grab and sample these pills (or at least the mush that those pills became). One health care worker was evidently too weary from the long trek to police his inventory, dropping supplies along the trail from riverbank to village. One curious small child, Demianus, uncapped a syringe and tried to peer closely at the needle only to poke it into his eye. He is now blind in that eye.

While we require patients to return on consecutive afternoons to our porch to complete multiday dosages, some health care workers have given a week's worth of medicine to some of the sick tribal locals who can neither read nor write. They either take too many or too little pills, or trade the pills to others. Good intentions are not enough when it comes to health care. We should never justify shoddy practices in the name of charity, "Do no harm" being the first cardinal rule by which we abide.

Pulong Banop, a Tribal Child Rescued From Death

When we first met Baby Pulong, her body was limp and feverish with both vivax and falciparum malaria (she was plus-4 for both according to laboratory tests on the coast). Malnourished, anemic, and stricken by trichuriasis (Whipworm) as well, her rectum was prolapsed and she suffered up to 30 bouts of foul mucus-filled diarrhea each day. Pulong was too weak to walk or stand, or even to sit unassisted.

Pulong's family lives in a remote treehouse over 8 hours to the West of my home in Danowage—a full day's walk and three river crossings away. Her mother knows only her tribal dialect and the outside world is frightening to her. There is a local belief that the world will end when the outside world intrudes upon the Korowai region. My mere presence is a harbinger of the Apocalypse.

I used my satellite phone to call for a medical evacuation by helicopter. Pulong's mother was terrified. Wild-eyed and screaming, she dashed into the jungle at the sight of the helicopter descending from the sky. We tried our best to explain the situation to her. Even then, she would not climb aboard. She handed over baby Pulong to our Christian coworker, Perin Lambe, from the highland Dani tribe. Desperate with grief and fear, Pulong's mother collapsed in the mud beside the trail as the heli lifted off.

Perin helped us care for Pulong in our home for the better part of the next year. Her malaria was cured (both kinds), her diarrhea disappeared, and the prolapsed rectum retracted. The lice were eradicated (after first spreading through my own household). Perin patiently helped us tend to the two-dozen episodes of explosive diarrhea a day. Finally, this, too, ceased and Pulong became stronger. Pulong learned first how to sit, stand, and then walk in our home. Suffering a jaw deformity, she only learned to talk with great difficulty. The sight on the face of Pulong's mother was of happy disbelief when Perin returned Pulong to her.

Two years later, we received a visitor from the jungle. It was Pulong. Instead of being carried limply in a net-bag, Pulong walked for 8 hours to my village along with her mother and father, her own small net-bag hanging from her head. They handed over a fish in gratitude.

Maltreatment of Papuans in City Hospitals

Interior Papuans are Black, Melanesian, and tribal. They are also generally poor (if we don't count the value of tribal hunting lands) and suffer from limited access to education. Most other Indonesians are brown-skinned and from Malay descent. They live mostly in Western Indonesia and along the more accessible coastal regions of Papua. Much inequality exists. While visiting Java, I've had Western Indonesians ask, "Do those Papuans have tails?" One Javanese doctor stationed (reluctantly it seems) at one Papuan hospital desired strongly to amputate one of our Papuan friend's feet after only a cursory examination and without first discussing any other options with the patient. His rationale: "Well, he's a tribal guy. They don't know much—the foot will just become infected anyhow, you know that these Papuans don't bathe much. It is best just to cut it off now."

I believe nurses have a moral obligation to advocate on behalf of their patients. The Bible demands: "*Speak up for those who cannot speak for themselves, for the rights of all who are destitute*" (Proverbs 31:8). Advocacy (even loud advocacy) is thus a divine imperative. When our coworker, Jimmy Weyato, was mauled by a pig and the bones in his toes were bitten through, amputation was also the first and only option considered. At least until two foreign nurses made a scene. We finally found a kind-hearted Christian doctor, a Javanese man who felt called by God to serve the medical needs of Papua. He took over Jimmy's care, operated before obtaining proof of any means of payment, discounted the fees when he learned of Jimmy's financial state, and placed steel rods to reposition toes that hung askew from the tusks of the attacking wild pig. Jimmy now plays soccer again just as before. He treks from jungle post to jungle post with me again, hours and hours on muddy jungle trail, just like before ("just like before," meaning barefoot).

Baby Sebideyos—Suctioned to Death by Careless Nursing

Sometimes the story does not end so well. We are always in a dilemma with difficult cases as to whether to treat the patient on-site (in our home) or send them out by heli to a bigger facility. Baby Sebideyos was Kesia and Yonas's first child and was suffering severely from respiratory syncytial virus (RSV). We improvised a croup tent with boiling water, Vicks VapoRub, and a plastic sheet, but we lacked oxygen or suction capabilities in our jungle post. Should we monitor Baby Sebideyos here, or should we send him out to the hospital in

Wamena? The mother knew but little of the national language or the outside world. Most people in my village have never even seen a car before.

We sent her out by heli medivac. Back in Danowage, we waited for results. The next day we learned the awful news. The nurse in Wamena had inserted the suction tube to help clear Baby Sebideyos' congestion . . . and then left it in at full suction for over a full minute without pause. Baby Sebideyos died mid-suction with the tube still inserted. The hospital staff then shifted blame to Kesia, who had tried to breast-feed Sebideyos to calm him on the heli flight to Wamena. "He choked on your milk," the hospital staff told Kesia. We transported the tiny body back to Danowage the next day. We would normally bury the dead in the city, but the father Yonas had threatened to shoot us with his bow and arrows if the baby died. When Kesia returned, she seemed to defend our care and calmed the feelings of Yonas. Then she began her several days of ritual wailing at her baby's death.

Cerebral Malaria and No Way to Evacuate

Ledipena started seizing at 5:30 a.m. She had been barely conscious most of the previous night after collapsing at the airstrip the previous afternoon. Ledipena is the wife of the highland church worker, Endiles, and they were together helping the local Korowai tribe continue their 5-year-long labor of carving out a dirt airstrip from dense jungle foliage using only simple tools and back-breaking work. Ledipena had been sick for 2 days prior and had barely eaten or drank during all that time.

We decided to medically evacuate her to the coast. Then we learned that the floatplane that services our village by landing on our river was experiencing mechanical issues and was not available. The helicopter that we often use for emergency medical evacuations was also disassembled for inspection. The weather was rainy and the river was flooded and only marginally safe for the full-day float down to Yaniruma by dugout canoe. She wasn't stable enough to tolerate that ride and the water was too choppy to safely transport someone who was not fully conscious. We felt trapped.

We started an IV and infused the World Health Organization (WHO) standard high loading dose of quinine for severe cerebral malaria. All day Tuesday and Wednesday her breathing was labored and she suffered occasional seizures. It looked several times as if she was beginning to decompensate. At one point we concluded that she seemed to be in the process of dying. The highland Dani Christians gathered around her bed and began to pray. Her breathing normalized again precisely as they prayed.

Early on Wednesday morning, we ran out of IV quinine and fluids. We normally stock enough meds for most cases of most sicknesses, and we had enough IV quinine and fluids to stabilize a patient in order to get the patient out to Wamena. But we did not have enough to keep and treat a critical patient locally for an extended period of time in the village without resupply.

Mission Aviation Fellowship came to the rescue. They flew slowly at treetop level over our village and chucked specially prepared padded boxes of meds and fluids out of the airplane window. These padded boxes thudded down in a perfect bull's-eye among the soft bushes near our simple church building (only two IV bags broke, but the rest of the meds were recovered intact). This allowed us to continue the quinine dosing and IV fluids for several more days.

Friday morning, Ledipena began to improve and follow us with her eyes. Then she began to cry for her children. We continued IV fluids, meds, and then progressed to oral rehydration with juice and then oatmeal through a nasogastric tube until she could began eating on her own. During episodes of anxiety my 6-year-old very blonde-headed son, Noah, would stand at the foot of her bed and smile, and Ledipena would immediately calm at his presence. The next week, she was able to walk by herself.

THE IMPACT OF WORLDVIEW AND CULTURE UPON HEALTH CARE

Culture may be defined loosely as those traits that make up a particular group of people (customs, rites, social practices). Culture would include things such as food and dress and music and language.

Worldview goes deeper. It focuses on the inner make-up of a person or group. Worldview (*weltanschauung*, if you prefer German) is a lens through which we see the entirety of reality. Whatever worldview we hold becomes a filter, a grid, through which we process the data from our senses. Our experiences of life and the moral and philosophical values we attach rightly or wrongly to reality are determined by whatever worldview we possess. Our worldview determines whether we suspect witchcraft when we fall sick, blame bad vapors, or attribute disease to germs.

Indulge me for just a second with this following mental exercise. Think about American cultural values. How do these American cultural values impact health, either for good or ill? How does belief (even religious belief) impact the following health care concerns in the West: heart disease, diabetes, obesity, sexually transmitted diseases, HIV/AIDS, addictions, abortion, and trauma from domestic abuse as well as child abuse? All of these health care concerns have deep psycho-social implications and are closely linked to lifestyle or life choices, which are closely linked to worldview.

As a nurse and a pastor, and one living overseas and keenly aware of the influence of culture on health care, I want to strongly assert that health care must not focus on the merely physical. We must ever be mindful of worldview when treating the sick and remember that we do not merely treat a physical body, but a human whole. We are not merely biological pieces of matter that sometimes go awry and need fixing. We are whole systems who have psycho-social, spiritual, and sexual components. In fact, the physical aspect is not even our most significant aspect. To summarize the theologians, we are not bodies possessing a soul, but the other way around. We are souls possessing a body. This most substantial part of us, the soul, is unable to be dissected by a surgical knife, subjected to lab exams, or seen under a microscope. If we dichotomize human beings and attempt to treat their biology without changing their habits and beliefs our success will be limited.

Being a Positive Change-Agent While Respecting Local Culture

Worldview changes lead to health changes. We desire to respect the local culture, even while serving as positive change-agents. Missionaries have a long history of impacting the health and well-being of local communities for the good. Baptist missionary William Carey helped end the brutal practice of Suttee in India (widow burning). Missionaries to Japan helped stop the foot-binding of Japanese women and helped advance their place in society. Until the 1970s, over half (some say nearly 75%) of all African schools were mission-run. William Wilberforce was a committed Christian who labored for decades to end the slave trade.

The sociologist Robert Woodberry more recently claimed in the article, "The Missionary Roots of Liberal Democracy," in the May 2012 issue of *American Political Science Review*, "The work of missionaries . . . turns out to be the single largest factor in insuring the health of nations." Woodberry continues on page 39, "Areas where Protestant missionaries had a significant presence in the past are on average more economically developed today, with comparatively better health, lower infant mortality, lower corruption, greater literacy, higher educational attainment (especially for women), and more robust membership in nongovernmental associations."

Our beliefs about God, the world, and reality must impact how we treat our fellow man. Our culture and worldview (including our spirituality) must have practical social implications. I am glad to be a missionary nurse because it allows me to address the whole person.

It is true that a careless approach to culture-change may result in unintended negative consequences for indigenous cultures. In an effort to end polygamy in Africa, some missionaries encouraged divorce for polygamous couples. In one fell swoop, this rendered many former wives destitute of material means of support and their children immediately changed in status and became "illegitimate" overnight because of careless mission policies. It is imperative for every missionary nurse to become a student of the culture that they are serving.

We desire to be positive change agents, but this does not mean that we desire to destroy indigenous cultures or become cultural imperialists. I want to see the end of witchcraft accusations. I seek the end of wife beating. I long for the extinction of tribal infanticide. I hope for the end of superstitious food taboos that steal vital protein intake away from pregnant and nursing mothers. I desire, however, in all of my efforts to preserve all that is noble and good about this culture. Each and every tribal person is a special creation of God, worthy of love and respect. Every human culture displays the glory of God's immeasurable variety and creativity.

ADVICE TO NURSES DESIRING TO SERVE OVERSEAS

What advice would I give somebody pursuing a nursing career in a cultural context not their own? Here is a short list: (1) Be flexible, (2) be open-minded, (3) invest in language and culture learning, (4) look for things that you absolutely love about your new culture (and remember those things on difficult days), (5) make lasting friendships with locals—they can be gentle cultural guides, (6) if you are having a bad day, just withdraw and have a stash of good American candy and movies for pure escapism, then jump right back on that horse and get to work again after such a break, (7) see each patient as a Creation of God, with unique value and dignity, (8) think longterm, (9) focus on disease prevention and health education over merely treating the recurring sick, (10) manage your expectations (sometimes this means "aim for the dirt and be happy with any results higher than that"), (11) take care of yourself and prevent your own physical breakdown lest you be no good to anybody else, (12) learn to disengage and vacation without allowing nagging thoughts about your place of duty to steal away your moments of relaxation (leave work at work).

A FINAL WORD

Though we live in a difficult area, we thank God every day that we can serve here. The quality of our lives is not to be judged by what we gather to ourselves, but by what we can give to others. We feel so very fortunate for the privilege of serving where we do.

II

Global Health Nursing as an Avocation

A Passion for Doing More

Nurses who already have very active lives and fulfilling careers describe how they responded to the call to work in settings very different from their everyday work world. These nurses have a passion to go above and beyond, to do more, and when opportunity knocked they seized the moment. In retrospect it seems that "Carpe diem: seize the day!" might have been a more appropriate title for this section.

10

Rising From the Ashes

Hospice, Health, and Holism in Sierra Leone

JACQUELINE BOULTON

Editor's Note: Jacqui Boulton teaches at the Florence Nightingale School of Nursing and Midwifery in London, and travels periodically to Sierra Leone where she provides consultation to a program offering hospice services. Sierra Leone is a country recovering from great conflict and genocide. Jacqui talks about her surprise that hospice would be a priority in a country faced with so many compelling problems. As she describes her work she weaves history and local beliefs into her narrative. A number of Brits, Jacqui included, are contributors to this work, so speakers of American English may notice an occasional British influence in word choice or phrasing. Enjoy the difference!

Dear Sir/Madam, I am currently in my third year of training to be a nurse and am interested in working in Sudan on completion. Please advise me how I go about this?

—My letter to Voluntary Services Overseas [VSO] some 30 years ago!

WHY GLOBAL HEALTH?

I cannot say what initially drew me toward working in global health. It may be a cliché, but it was always in me. A colleague recently mentioned to me that, in her experience, those who are attracted to global health fall into one of four categories: heartbroken, desirous of an expat lifestyle, unable to fit in their own society, or having a desire to change the world. I am not sure I entirely agree, but I do recognize it was probably the latter which prompted my interest as a naive 20 year old. I have come to realize that this motivation alone cannot be sustained for long when up against the realities of life in the field.

I was rather put out that the letter I wrote to Voluntary Services Overseas did not elicit a wholly positive response, including how grateful they were for my kind offer and when would I like to start! Rather, the advice given was to get more experience and training and, in particular, a midwifery qualification.

PREPARATION AND PATIENCE

Despite feeling a little affronted that my offer to work in Sudan was not greeted with open arms, I took the advice seriously and enrolled in a midwifery program. I also met my future husband and fell in love! I struggled with the choice between marriage and an overseas adventure. My husband-to-be was in the process of establishing himself in a financial career, and in those days it didn't seem proper to get married and leave him "home alone." So I determined to settle down to married life, gain experience, and put my ambitions on hold until later. "Later" came when my children were 12 and 15. By then I had worked as a nurse in neurology, as a midwife, as a cardiology research nurse, and as a practice nurse gaining additional qualifications in contraception and sexual health, health needs assessment, and asthma management. With the children at secondary school, it was now time to pursue my own goals again. I enrolled in the excellent diploma in Tropical Nursing at the London School of Hygiene and Tropical Medicine, which is a program for nurses and midwives with course content similar to a master's degree in public health (MPH). Doors open in unexpected ways, and shortly after I had an opportunity to visit The Shepherd's Hospice (TSH) in Sierra Leone. The visit was initiated by Sheila Hurton—founder of Voices for Hospices, which organizes a worldwide series of concerts every 2 years on World Hospice and Palliative Care Day. This series of concerts raises funds and awareness for hospice work, including TSH in Sierra Leone (Voices of Hospices, 2013).

After completing the diploma in Tropical Nursing, I sought advice from its director about other qualifications that may be useful to my interests in global health and went on to complete an MSc in Medical Anthropology. This included a further period in Sierra Leone, undertaking a research project about the socioeconomic, political, and cultural influences on the hospice model. I also was offered a post at the Florence Nightingale Faculty of Nursing & Midwifery, Kings College London and completed a teaching qualification. I now have the privilege of leading the Global Health Module for nursing students and of supporting them in undertaking international electives. I am also involved with the Health Partnerships at Kings Centre for Global Health (Kings Centre for Global Health 2013). I recently spent a short period in Somaliland in conjunction with the Kings/THET/Somaliland project looking at the issues and challenges facing nursing and midwifery in the country. I also represent nursing on the management committee of the newly formed King's Sierra Leone partnership.

The focus of this chapter will be my ongoing involvement, both directly and indirectly, with the work of TSH in Sierra Leone.

SIERRA LEONE: THE IMPORTANCE OF HISTORY

Any nurse wishing to work trans-nationally should begin by researching the context of their planned setting as broadly as possible. This is essential groundwork in helping to understand and appreciate the many challenges and differences that are likely to arise. Sierra Leone is still classified as a fragile and conflict-affected state, which requires some difficult reading. Sierra Leone is about the size of Ireland; numerically its population is around 20% larger at 5,612,685, but its population profile and life expectancy is vastly different (Central Intelligence Agency [CIA] 2013). It was discovered in 1460 by Pedra de Cinta, a Portuguese explorer, who named it Sierra Lyoa, meaning Lion Mountain. It later became the first settlement for rescued slaves, hence the name of its capital Freetown. In 1807 it became a crown colony, was placed under British Protectorate in 1896, and gained independence in 1961. Six years later a series of military coups began, eventually leading to a vicious and bloody civil war between 1991 and 2002. Events reached their peak on January 6, 1999, with a devastating surge on Freetown known as "Operation No Living Thing." During a 3-week period, 6,000 people lost their lives and some 150,000 were displaced. Eventually peace was reinstated with the help of the United Nations and elections have subsequently been held.

THE SHEPHERD'S HOSPICE

I first met Mr. Gabriel Madiye, founder and director of TSH, in 2001 when I was a student in Tropical Nursing. He visited my church and spoke of his attempts to establish a hospice in Freetown and the desecration of two previous hospice sites during the war. He also alluded to his own personal suffering.

While inspired I was also surprised, since the whole notion of hospice seemed to be at odds with the African context. My understanding of the concept was as a Western reaction against the increasing medicalization of death and dying (Illich, 1960). I could not imagine medicalization being an issue in what was then, according to the United Nations Human Development Report, the poorest country in the world. In addition, I had heard many accounts about extended family systems; legendary tales in which everyone seemed to be related to everyone else. I therefore assumed that the social structure of African societies would guard against the isolation so often experienced by the dispersion of family relationships in the United Kingdom. In addition, I found it difficult to understand the rationale for founding a hospice in a country trying to recover from a lengthy and horrific civil war and therefore drowning in all kinds of other needs.

It was now 2004, several years since I had met Mr. Madiye and just 2 years since the conflict had ended. Even with the questions raised by his earlier talk, I was keen to accept Sheila Hurton's invitation to accompany her on a visit to Sierra Leone. I was also apprehensive. Was it safe? How would I cope with the sight of so many people, and in particular of children, who had been maimed and mutilated as a result of the conflict? Amputation of limbs and other body parts had been common during the war; those involving the arm were referred to by the perpetrators as short sleeve above the elbow . . . or long sleeve, anywhere below. In this context, could I be of any use?

My background and skills are very broad but I had no specific expertise in palliative care. I was greatly relieved to learn that Ruth Cecil, a community nurse specialist in palliative care and current chair of the UK Friends of the Shepherd's Hospice (UKFTSH), would also be joining our team. I found myself heading to Sierra Leone with absolutely no idea of what to expect, although I did know there would be no electricity and no running water. We had been asked to develop a 2-day workshop to train nurses working at the hospice and in partner institutions throughout Freetown. I wanted to make sure I was as well prepared as possible, with rolls of wallpaper for flip charts and bags and bags of pens donated by various drug companies. I also packed items to protect our own health and safety: sterilizing tablets and charcoal filters in case bottled water was not available.

One of my first impressions was of the number of people in wheelchairs with skinny limbs, which I later learned was a result of polio. During civil war, survival becomes the name of the game—neither vaccines nor education are a priority!

Both Ruth and I were determined that our teaching be relevant. Since we had no experience in that environment, we insisted that we spend time working alongside the team, observing home visits by nurses and social workers, attending clinics at the hospice, eating and conversing over breakfast and lunch, sitting in on meetings, and visiting other relevant facilities and agencies. It felt important to try to understand the challenges facing our colleagues. During this observation phase, our days began around 6:30 a.m. with a candlelight breakfast—there was, and still is, very limited electricity in Sierra Leone. Walking around as the "lady with the lamp" seemed particularly poignant given that I was now employed at the Florence Nightingale Faculty of Nursing & Midwifery. After breakfast, we travelled to the hospice to spend our day with various team members (two nurses, one community medical officer, and two social workers). I had assumed the hospice would be an inpatient facility, but learned that the model is home-based care. A walk-in clinic also operates 6 days a week. Generally, we made the return journey home around 6:00 p.m., engaging in further conversation over supper with whoever happened to be around before retiring to make notes and make plans for our workshop. Any nurse planning to work "in the field" should remember that it is vital to keep notes on a daily basis, no matter how tired you may feel. You never know what might turn out to be significant!

Based on our observations and discussions we devised a teaching plan we hoped would be relevant. We tried to factor in a degree of flexibility now that we had a clearer idea about what we wanted to cover. However, our timetable, and Western mindset, were somewhat disrupted by the inclusion of breakfast (which was an important "incentive" to encourage attendance), an opening ceremony, daily prayer, and lengthy words of thanks! Our teaching methodology included group work, feedback, and role play. We felt these strategies would help determine levels of understanding and practice upon which we could build in the future. Such interactive learning, however, is not the norm in Sierra Leone, where teaching is mainly didactic in its approach. As with any group of people, some participants took more easily to this new style of learning than others. One of our main foci was, and continues to be, on the importance of record keeping. We brought examples of initial assessment documents with us in hopes of adapting them to the Sierra Leone context. One of the assessment questions asked about religion and there was a tick box for "none." The "none" category caused great concern among the participants. The idea that anyone might say they did not have a religion was clearly a complete anathema.

We planned to include role play on breaking bad news, but we learned that addressing such concerns is not readily done in Sierra Leone. While this is still the case, it is a skill that the hospice team has adopted and in which they continue to receive training. Since our initial training, a number of nurses and community health officers have been supported, through UKFTSH and the African Palliative Care Association to participate in palliative care training at Hospice Uganda.

We learned something new too! The team introduced us to an important method of their own: a number of "sensitization" songs they wrote to get the message across. Because literacy rates are quite low, the use of songs and drama (TSH now has its own touring drama group) is therefore vital in contributing to "sensitization" and the reduction of stigma surrounding sickness, particularly HIV/AIDS and cancer.

ON UNDERSTANDING AND BEING UNDERSTOOD

Many nurses who engage with global health projects outside their own country of residence will need to learn a different language. In Sierra Leone, English is the official language but its use is primarily limited to the literate minority. In Freetown, English-based Creole is understood by most patients and spoken by the majority. Conversing with the nurses at TSH has generally not been a problem. Nevertheless, extreme concentration was required at times to cut through accents. One particularly amusing example stands out.

On a visit to the Christian Health Association of Sierra Leone (CHASL), one of the nurses pointed out a gentleman who she said had been her teacher in nursing school.

"What did he teach you?" I asked. "Mending hats," came the reply. Somewhat surprised, I asked again and got the same response.

Anxious to overcome any preconceived ideas I may have inherited about the appropriate content of nurse training, I tried to convince myself that, for some reason, this must be an important part of the curriculum in Sierra Leone. I could not, however, quite bring myself to leave it there and decided to try and resolve things one more time. "Just tell me one more time. What did that man teach you?" "Mending hats," she replied, and suddenly I understood. "Oh, you mean mending hearts!" I was familiar with this phrase from billboards offering the postwar counseling services of numerous international nongovernmental organizations.

THE NEED FOR A JOINED-UP APPROACH

Concepts of global health increasingly recognize a need for a "joined-up approach," in other words, a collaborative approach. Nobody can wave a magic wand in any given situation, but interventions will be much more successful if they also seek to challenge and change the existing context. In the decade since my first visit to Sierra Leone, there have been some very significant improvements in the country. Nevertheless, the underlying context of extreme poverty in which staff and patients coexist influences both the ability of staff to provide care and the capacity of patients to receive it.

For the patients, the bitter challenge of everyday life has major implications on their ability to absorb the health education they receive during home visits and clinic sessions. For example, one of the patients I visited, who I will call Victoria, had recently been diagnosed HIV positive and was now quite unwell, with a series of opportunistic infections resulting from full-blown AIDS. Victoria had three young children and worked as a commercial sex worker. When she was well enough, she continued to go to work. Although the hospice provides free condoms—donated by Standard Charter Bank—Victoria explained that she would be less well paid or more probably would not get work at all if she tried to use them. Her priority and those of her coworkers was the need for everyday sustenance rather than concerns about contracting or spreading a disease that might kill them in years to come.

Another patient, whom I will call Earnest, was unable to rest his severely swollen left leg as we recommended. The edema was caused by lymphoedema—a mark of his advanced HIV status. Given his condition, it was surprising to find he had gone out when

I accompanied Christine on a visit to his house. Despite having to use a crutch to negotiate the currently dry river bed that meandered from his house to the main road, he had gone to town to ask his brother (the only relative who had not disowned him) for money to buy food. Although the patient support fund assists with nutritional support for those on its books, it is not enough.

COMBATING STIGMA

Most palliative care patients who receive care from TSH are HIV/AIDS positive and/or suffer from cancer. Both of these conditions are usually not diagnosed until they are quite advanced. In the past, this has been due to a combination of lack of diagnostics and lack of treatment. While these issues remain (for example, no histology or intravenous chemotherapy is available), there have been some positive developments, including improved access to antiretroviral medications, and for the first time oral morphine (International Association of Palliative Care, 2009).

My most significant and surprising discovery is the overwhelming societal stigma with which HIV/AIDS seems to be regarded. It is difficult to understand why this should be the case, given the conditions for its spread, including poverty, polygamy, and rape, are common.

The impact on patients I visited was always apparent and caused a plethora of emotions. I recall visiting Thomas, a 24-year-old man who had just completed his university education. In other ways, his story was quite typical. Thomas had been suffering from prolonged bouts of ill health for several years and had paid for a number of blood tests, but nothing was found. He had finally agreed to an HIV test, which was positive. He was living with his mother and five sisters in a dark brick-built building with a number of corridors and separate rooms leading off them. He had not revealed his diagnosis to his family. "They would throw me onto the street," he said. The nurses had asked in advance if he would mind if I accompanied them during one of their visits. Apparently he was very happy with that, as he thought I would be able to provide antiretroviral therapy. Unlike the uneducated majority, he was aware of the existence of such medication and was very angry that it was not available to him. Sadly, Thomas died 4 months later.

I always expect to see difficult sights during home care visits, but a recent visit to see a patient in the main hospital in Freetown who had been referred to TSH stands out. As we walked through a very large ward it became apparent that the patient we had been called to see, whom I will call Isata, was in the far corner shrouded by a curtain. On navigating through the curtain I was met with one of the most disturbing and confusing sights I have ever come across: a skeletal and dyspnoeic lady sitting up on a bare mattress. The characteristic marks of Kaposi's sarcoma pointed to end-stage AIDS, which was the apparent reason for the screen. She had no access to water, and although physically occupying a bed, a note at the end of the bed indicated she had been discharged 2 days ago! In other words, they had withdrawn care. Isata had been abandoned by the relatives who had brought her to the hospital. The patient support fund was used to buy two sheets, a pillow, water, and food. The priority for TSH was to reinvolve her relatives and encourage them to take her home. After some impressive detective work, a nurse and a social worker managed to track down her aunt, and after much discussion persuaded Isata's family to take her home. In doing so, TSH promised to visit every other day, pay for an ambulance to transfer her, and provide some rice. Isata died peacefully in her home village, a very different scenario to that which would have occurred without the intervention of TSH.

HEALTH BELIEFS

Health beliefs, theories about disease causation, and widespread myths influence the type of treatment accessed by those who are sick as well as their attitude toward prevention. The context in which TSH operates is infused with differing notions, particularly in relation to HIV/AIDS and cancer. The following story highlights the widely held belief in witchcraft that I encountered on a number of occasions. The conversation was with the wife of a late patient who had been referred to TSH but had subsequently died. She had her 8-year-old daughter with her, and in hushed tones, told me that at the end "his legs were very bad." I asked her if she knew what caused his illness.

He was shot with a witch gun. Do you know it?

No. They tried to remove the bullet from his knee but they could not find it.

Although my initial thoughts were that a "witch gun" may be some sort of curse, this talk of surgery and removing bullets made me think I was jumping to false conclusions.

So what does a witch gun look like?

It is a witch gun. (I now realize this was rather a naïve question.)

Could you draw it for me?

No, you do not see it.

So is it like a real gun?

No, it is not a real gun.

But you mention the bullet. Was there a bullet there?

Well, they could not find it.

So who might carry such a gun?

They are evil men and they come out at night. It is very powerful. It is a witch gun and if you are shot you will die in 20 to 30 days. (Her explanation was very earnest.)

Later that evening I mentioned this to Mr. Madiye, who said, "Oh yes I too saw her today. She had a boyfriend. He was HIV positive and we offered him support but they decided to drive him up to Kenema where he died." As already mentioned, by the time many patients are diagnosed, their illness is quite advanced. Most first seek help from witch doctors, herbalists, or religious healers. This often happens and, frustratingly, may well impede the care offered by TSH.

On another occasion, while looking at the issues and challenges of treating patients with oral morphine, we visited a patient with Kaposi's sarcoma. He mentioned having attended a funeral recently and seemed evasive. We later learned that he had left town to visit a witch doctor back home.

I also recall sitting in on a conversation with relatives of a patient with fungating breast cancer. They brought her for treatment because of the smell, and were reluctant to care for her at home. The staff spent much time persuading the family that they could not catch the cancer, and with the offer of ongoing support—and the realization that an inpatient facility was not an option—they agreed to take her home.

I've given several examples from patient encounters, but it is important to recognize that our colleagues, even if their training was based on Western biomedical concepts, are also products of their own culture. They may give textbook answers, but occasionally deep-seated beliefs will come through, affording interesting insights regarding health beliefs. For example, while chatting with one of the hospice nurses, I was taken by surprise when she casually mentioned:

After the war there was a lot of liver cancer.

Really? (My medically trained mind immediately starts racing to see if I can think of any obvious connection or reason why this might make sense).

Yes, the rebels came out of the bush and they all had liver cancer. They had big swollen here (points under the ribs)—*a curse had been put on them because of their cannibalism.*

The conversation then reverted back to the point at which it had been sidetracked and I tried to disguise my amazement.

COMPETING PRIORITIES AMONG NGOs AND DONOR-LED AGENCIES

Prior to my first visit to Sierra Leone, I assumed that TSH's primary work would be to maintain and administer an inpatient facility. In fact, I visited a quite large facility. However, there were apparently only four beds and somehow the assertion that they were indeed used for hospice care was unconvincing. Certainly I saw no evidence of it. Perhaps things were just a bit quiet. I would have to bide my time to see if I could work out what was going on and, more importantly, why. After a number of gentle enquiries, comments, and observations, the reality of the situation emerged. It became apparent that the tendency for Western donors to assume that their own successful models of care should be adopted was at work. The need for an inpatient facility was largely determined by one of the major donors. The idea of inpatient care was never accepted by the hospice staff themselves, who preferred home-based care. Three main reasons were given for this. Firstly, it was felt that, given the stigma already discussed, an inpatient facility would simply become a dumping ground. Secondly, safety for hospice staff and patients was a concern. A number of incidents had occurred of spitting and throwing stones at patients. Thirdly, the additional cost of providing round-the-clock nursing care was prohibitive. As I write the tide is turning. Funding has been secured to begin construction on a new inpatient facility. However, much work needs to be done to assure acceptance of this new health care delivery system on the part of staff, patients, families, and the larger community.

THE VALUE OF EXPERIENCE IN GLOBAL HEALTH NURSING

Experience in global health nursing offers many transferrable skills. It teaches you to think outside the box. It heightens the ability to critically analyze, encourages resilience, and above all, promotes the important nursing concepts of empowering others to take responsibility for their own health and advocating for the health needs of those who are disempowered. These are universal skills needed both at home and abroad, for increasingly in our globalized societies they have become us.

REFERENCES

Central Intelligence Agency. (2013). *World fact book*. Retrieved December 20, 2013, from https://www.cia.gov/library/publications/the-world-factbook/geos/sl.html

Illich, I. (1976). *Limits to Medicine.* Marion Boyars.

King's College London. (2013). *Kings Center for global health*. Retrieved December 2013, from http://www.kcl.ac.uk/aboutkings/worldwide/initiatives/global/global-health/partnerships/index.aspx

World Hospice and Palliative Care Day. (2013). *Voices for hospices*. Retrieved December 2013, from http://www.worldday.org/voices-for-hospices/

11

Resilience and Recovery

Mental Health Care in Postconflict Rwanda

CAROLE F. BENNETT

Editor's Note: Carole Bennett demonstrates that even toward the end of a fulfilling career there is energy and desire to make a difference in a new way. Carole seized the opportunity to travel to Rwanda where she joined Marie Donahue (Chapter 1) and Tina Anselmi-Moulaye (Chapter 2) and contributed toward rebuilding the mental health services infrastructure. Like Sierra Leone (Chapter 10), Rwanda is also recovering from great tragedy with enormous mental health implications. Carole approached her assignment with grace and resourcefulness as she sought practical solutions to problems encountered.

As a teenage candy striper, I quickly discovered that I loved being in the hospital and watching nurses' intimate involvement in peoples' lives. I thought that what they did mattered, and in one short day I was sure that I would commit my life to being a nurse. My career has included work with inmates in prisons, with adolescents in hospitals, program development for pregnant drug-addicted women, and day treatment for small children. My career has been meaningful and satisfying. However, after being a registered nurse for 44 years and an advanced practice registered nurse (APRN) for 40 years, having practiced psychiatric nursing in all areas of mental health care, I was ready for a new challenge.

AFRICA BOUND

My adult children are now working, scattered across the world. It is their lives that give me inspiration. And so it was, that at a time when I could have retired, and although I have never worked and rarely travelled outside of the United States, I headed to Africa.

I found myself on a crowded bus as it pushed through motos and pedestrians winding its way through roundabouts, through crowded streets, to Ndera Psychiatric Hospital, high on a hill on the outskirts of Kigali. The bus as well as the hospital belonged to the Brothers of Charity, who had founded it and other psychiatric hospitals in Africa in the 1970s. Hoards of people streaming by, motos hovering and then suddenly bursting forth like swarms of bees, I had never imagined anything like what I was seeing. Little did I know then that this would be the beginning of only one of several phases of my work in Africa.

It had all happened very quickly. Within 10 days, I finished up my teaching job, packed with the help of my daughter who was visiting from Morocco, piled onto a plane, and was on my way to Rwanda. I had been assigned to work at the only psychiatric hospital in the country, and with some trepidation, my adventure began. With a PhD some would say I was overqualified, but with my meager travel experience and lack of any language besides English, my confidence wavered to say the least.

What was clear to me right away was that the people who were with me on the bus and who worked together at the hospital were happy to see one another and to be going to work together. Although I couldn't understand what they were saying, I could see their loving attention to one another. If someone who was expected failed to show up at a bus stop, cell phones came out, calls were made, and the bus waited. They poked fun at one another lovingly, and even the person who was being ridiculed laughed uproariously with everyone else on the bus. At times they burst into song, singing hymns harmonized beautifully in minor keys, obviously memorized from years of mass and training in catechism. The presence of the Catholic Church was strongly felt. This was their life and they appeared to be a grateful and warm people.

PHASE 1: CLINICAL CARE AT NDERA HOSPITAL

As we came through the gate, I saw a series of brightly painted one-story stucco buildings, connected by long covered walkways.

The buildings were surrounded by well-kept African gardens with flowering trees and swarms of brightly colored sunbirds. It looked welcoming, even comforting. It wasn't long, however, before cries and shrieks were heard of patients too ill to be calmed even in this serene place.

The woman I had been assigned to work with greeted me. She spoke some English and had a bachelor's of science (BS) degree in nursing. She had the kindest face I thought I had ever seen. It was because of her strengths and language skills that I was asked to work with her. I soon found out that these qualifications also made it necessary for her to travel to meetings and trainings all over the country. Unfortunately, she was rarely at the hospital and I would find myself with long days and no one to talk to who could speak English.

I found that what I could do was read one or two columns of the volumes and volumes of blue books; patient ledgers that the nursing staff wrote in laboriously hour after hour, day after day. Although they were written in French, I could decipher whether the patient had a previous hospitalization, what district he or she was from, and eventually the diagnosis. Therefore, almost immediately, I knew that their rate of rehospitalization was approximately 72%, the diagnosis of substance abuse was 25% of the male population in the hospital who were mostly diagnosed with brief psychosis, and rarely did I see the diagnosis of PTSD (posttraumatic stress disorder), which was reported to be 37% in the population in the years following the 1994 genocide. These discoveries made me curious. I also discovered, with the use of a map of Rwanda, that most hospitalized patients were from the local district, with patients occasionally being admitted from outlying districts. This made me wonder what, if any, services were available in these rural districts. Knowing there were people there with mental illnesses, I wondered about their care.

The conditions at the hospital were brutal, with overcrowding being the most obvious problem; the approximately 250-bed hospital was at an almost constant 160% capacity with two patients to a bed, which was actually a small cot. There was no safe running water. There were no bed sheets except for small blankets for covering. The sewer connected to a series of outhouses was situated close to the patients' sleeping areas. The sharp smell of the sewer constantly permeated the air.

I was anxious to learn more and, after asking for help, was assigned a nurse who could speak English to assist me. He did not have a BS degree in nursing but was more available and wanted the opportunity to work with me. We worked well together. I decided that I needed to interview patients in order to understand why so many people were readmitted, and why there was lack of information regarding the 1994 genocide in the patients' history.

Each day Manuel and I interviewed two or three male patients in a small office with a desk and three chairs. Patients were eager to be interviewed and answered my questions willingly. Even though I didn't speak their language, I looked directly at the patient while speaking the question to Manual. They would look at him as he interpreted the question into their language—Kinyarwanda with some Swahili here and there. But once they began to answer their questions, they looked directly at me with searing intensity. While I couldn't understand their words until he interpreted for me, I could see they told their story with great feeling and were very eager to have the opportunity to talk about their life. They never stammered or hesitated. The story spilled out in a steady stream as though they had just held it in too long, and once started no longer could hold it back.

I was sensitive to the unspoken rule of not mentioning the genocide (the staff would mention "the war"), and I would simply ask, "Where were you in 1994?" Followed by, "What did you see?" I quickly learned that their lives had been a narrative of trauma, war, and displacement. Many had witnessed their parent's murder and some had been compelled to participate in the killing as children. Some parents died in refugee camps of disease or brothers were killed in refugee camps because they were thought to have been part of the militia. By now, most had returned to their home village but lacked adequate work, were at conflict with their extended family, and used alcohol and traditional healers to cope with living. They didn't return to Ndera for follow-up appointments because the travel took 1 month's pay and, therefore, they were unable to continue their outpatient care. Some had been in and out of the hospital for years.

The hospital administrator realized I was interviewing patients and sent for me. He had a list of people who had been in the hospital for as many as 4 years and he did not know why. They had been given names like Anonymous I, II, III, and he wanted me to interview them and report back to him. I discovered that many of these patients had a brain injury of some sort. What I now surmise, after visiting district hospitals, is that they were brought to a district hospital probably following a motor vehicle accident, with incoherent speech and brain swelling. They were given a psychiatric diagnosis incorrectly. No one knew their names; the patients did not recover their memory. However, they survived the brain injury and were soon transferred to the psychiatric hospital where they remained, their identity unknown.

However, with close questioning, some were able to reveal early memories, and with local knowledge and effective sleuthing I felt certain their home village could be identified.

One tragic situation I uncovered was that some families simply didn't want to be responsible for a mentally disabled family member. With no hope of recovery, these relatives were viewed as ravenous persons who would eat all of the food in their modest home, leaving none for a family who were already malnourished and starving. When parents died, the remaining siblings often did not have the resources to continue to feed and care for their disabled family member who was often mute, poorly managed, and misunderstood.

Another group of patients who had been in the hospital for an extended period were people who were hospitalized while living briefly in Rwanda but were exiled from Burundi, Kenya, or Congo. It was assumed they were fleeing some local conflict and the path of repatriation was uncertain. Apparently, going through the proper channels required significant documentation—which was daunting, lengthy, and time consuming. There was not an expedited method even if the patient was willing to return to his or her native country. Being mentally ill left them vulnerable in too many ways to be discharged without a plan for returning to a home.

I eventually realized that being a refugee in exile had become for many a way of life. During their exile, they made friends, started businesses, and sometimes married. Their lives were a mix of here and there, traveling back and forth, bundles piled high with children tied on backs, to visit family, move herds, and attend weddings or funerals. People didn't seem to question this nomadic existence. I suppose there are not many generations separating these people from their ancestors whose lives often crossed artificial geographical borders imposed by others.

Using the results of these interviews, I made a nursing assessment tool and a nursing acuity scale. I hoped to identify issues at admission and thereby reduce overcrowding by expediting discharge. Each physician made rounds weekly on 80 people. They did not have a system of determining who was improving other than by interviewing the patient. This was done by asking the patient—in a room of charts, nurses seated along a very long table, the doctor in the center—a series of seemingly unrelated and confusing questions. The patient sat in a chair on the other side of the table—in the middle of the room—alone. It looked more like an interrogation and seemed to me an ineffective method for determining if the patient was ready to go home, thus the long hospitalizations and the backlog for discharge.

I was hopeful that the tools could give important, needed information on admission about the patient's history and condition and then identify which patients had adequately improved and were ready for discharge. These were translated into French using Google Translate and edited by my capable assistant. I began a series of in-service programs to help staff learn the purpose and use of these tools. Manuel had implemented the acuity scale on the men's non-acute unit and the doctor spoke in booming, approving tones about the experience. However, in spite of their promises and affirmative nods, as I looked across this sea of faces, their expressions told me that they did not understand what I was saying, even with an interpreter. A real sense of the gulf that lay between us began to sink into my consciousness. This simply wasn't going to happen, in spite of my efforts, my tears, my admonitions and their smiles, and nods, and promises. They did not have experience with the process of change. In spite of government planning, the U.S. universities, and the good intentions of everyone involved, nothing was going to happen to change this machine that turned slowly at a pace and with a process they understood.

It was clear I needed to find another way to contribute to mental health care. I had many questions. How could a rural country develop a system of care that began in villages and, connected to a vast network of mental health nurses and community health workers, focus on prevention and rehabilitation with less emphasis on acute care and more offerings of services closer to home for those who needed it?

PHASE 2: TEACHING AT KIGALI HEALTH INSTITUTE

I had already been introduced to nursing students and faculty at Kigali Health Institute where Mental Health Nursing was taught as an advanced diploma. Nursing education in Rwanda is quite different than that in the United States. In East Africa, nurses all take year 1 together. Then at the beginning of year 2, the students are either placed in a midwifery program, general nursing, or mental health nursing. The mental health nursing program was developed on the campus of Ndera Hospital in the first years after the 1994 genocide and students were prepared to work in an acute care setting. In 2008, the students were moved to the Kigali Health Institute campus and their curriculum was broadened. Mental health services were being opened in district hospitals and students were taught both acute care and community mental health.

In East Africa, the rate of epilepsy is quite high and assumed to be a result of birth hypoxia. Over 50% of births in Rwanda are not attended by health care personnel. In communities, mental health nurses provide care to people with epilepsy as well as psychiatric illness. Therefore, the role of the mental health nurse in the community was to manage people with neurological illness as well as mental illness.

I had already begun to work with students and faculty from Kigali Health Institute during their clinical rotations at Ndera Hospital. So when they asked me to teach a course in psychiatric emergencies, I gladly accepted. Although I had only 2 weeks to prepare, the students in the course were completing a clinical rotation at Ndera and I had been holding post conferences with them. Using the assessment tool I had developed, I enumerated to them the specific psychiatric emergencies we would be learning to manage. I directed them to take the assessment tool, find a patient who had had a psychiatric emergency, and interview them using the tool in order to present the case to the class when they started the upcoming course. I could see they were uncomfortable with this assignment and lobbied to work in groups. They had this lobbying process well developed but I was firm. I reminded them that they would be graduating soon and working independently. For that reason I insisted they interview a patient alone as well as develop their presentation by themselves. Then I set about developing my lectures for the course.

I had learned that people in Rwanda do not speak English as well as I had been led to believe. A suggestion was made to give students material in writing so that as they listened while I spoke, they could understand better. I then tried to develop bilingual slides, which I am sure anyone who teaches in Africa soon discovers. With Google Translate open on my computer, I could pull up the slide with side-by-side text boxes, type in the left box, and cut and paste the text into Google Translate. The French words would immediately pop up on the right side, and I would cut and paste the French translation into the slide text box 2. In this way, I could teach them about mental illnesses, brain regions, specific neurotransmitters that had been changed by the illness, how they changed, and what medications did to return the brain and neurotransmitters to normal.

I used as many images of the brain as I could find. The students were transfixed. Rwandan faculty members generously read over my slides; the funniest translation glitch was for "eating and sleeping" the Google program had translated those words into "hotels and restaurants." However, Google Translate must have improved as time went on. Eventually I wouldn't even have anyone edit the slides. If the translation was not quite right, students were kind enough to overlook the mistakes and learn what I had intended.

After each lecture, selected students presented their patient interviews. We then discussed diagnosis, nursing care, and changes in the brain and the effect of medication and treatment. The next morning, I gave them a "pop test," which was a similar case to the one that had been presented the day before, including symptoms and neurotransmitters. After the test, we reviewed the questions as a group. The effect was that each psychiatric emergency and case was reviewed four times: the presentation, the discussion, the pop quiz, and the quiz review. The students really were engaged and performed extremely well on the final exam. I was amazed at their commitment.

The obstacles students have to overcome are numerous. First, there are no real textbooks assigned to the course. Although the students have computers, they are usually reconditioned computers that have been purchased and provided by the government. However, many do not have access to the Internet while off campus. There were not enough classrooms to accommodate all of the classes; therefore each Friday, the head of the school decided which classes would meet the following week and announced their location. The street noise was deafening in the class rooms, and while there was a blackboard, which leaned against the wall, writing on it was impossible; the surface irregular and the writing therefore illegible. In spite of these obstacles, the students really did learn about the brain and were very appreciative of the material presented.

The students I taught were next assigned to work at a district hospital to learn concepts of community mental health. I was very curious to answer my questions regarding mental health care in the rural areas. When we arrived, we were able to see the three psychiatric patients who were currently hospitalized. I looked forward to having my questions answered. As we visited the patients, my heart sank lower and lower. All three patients, as far as I could tell through the language barrier and inability to read the chart, had delirium and were not what in my country would be identified as psychiatric patients. They had suffered either closed-head injury from trauma, sepsis with high fever, or long bone fractures from presumably a vehicular accident. It was really at that moment that it became clear to me that the problems in the health care and education systems were complex and multilayered. I felt lost as though I could not find my place.

PHASE 3: POLICY DEVLOPMENT AT THE MINISTRY OF HEALTH

During the time I was teaching, I met the nurse in Rwanda who had responsibility for leadership in mental health nursing. As we talked about what was needed in Rwanda, a similar understanding emerged about the role of nurses in mental health care both in acute and community settings. When we realized the mutual synergy, we were very excited about working together to improve mental health care in the entire country. I began meeting with him weekly, was given assignments, and worked diligently to complete my assignments. First, I tackled writing standards of care for the country. The Council for Health Service Accreditation of Southern Africa (COHSASA) standards were given to me as a template. After having worked at Ndera Hospital and having visited a district hospital, I found that adapting the 12 standards to the Rwandan context was not difficult. We met weekly to review progress.

At the same time, as luck would have it, a physician who is married to a nurse midwife in my program was hired by the United Nations High Commission for Refugees (UNHCR) to manage health care in refugee camps in Rwanda. We began meeting with him monthly to determine what could be done to offer services at the refugee camp location. We hoped to lessen the burden on local hospitals, which were dealing with multiple emergencies because preventive services were not available. Through a series of meetings, a screening tool was developed for refugees to determine who needed immediate services: those who had had previous hospitalizations or had taken psychotropic medications regularly, those who had been sexually assaulted or otherwise traumatized during the conflict from which they were fleeing, those who were substance abusers and needed preventive care, and those who were suicidal and felt isolated and alienated. A plan was devised to train community health workers to intervene with the refugees who screened positive and offer services with supervision by a mental health nurse. This nurse would also serve as a liaison between the district hospital and the refugee camp, supervising community health workers and offering services through the hospital for those who needed a higher level of care. The plan was ambitious and will take a great deal of cooperation to implement, but the wheels were turning and the screening tool was being piloted as I departed the country.

As this book goes to press, there are a couple of projects that remain in process. Several months before I left, the nurse who is the chair for the Mental Health Nursing department asked me to write a guide for two mental health nursing courses. Because the lack of text books had been a significant obstacle, I felt this was an opportunity I needed to take advantage of. Using the World Health Organization (WHO) Mental Health Intervention Guide and the COHSASA Standards of Care as relevant and available resources, I wrote a basic 8-week course, which included for each week a PowerPoint lecture, important text with principles of care, and integration exercises for the students. Each week was introduced with an African aphorism to emphasize relevant African wisdom and current data about the prevalence of each psychiatric illness. The second, more advanced course was also presented in an 8-week format with PowerPoint lectures, text, and integration exercises. Each topic addressed issues of importance to an identified African vulnerable population such as refugees, chronic mentally ill in rural areas, orphans of HIV/AIDS, women who were victims of gender-based violence, pregnant women and children, and incarcerated mentally ill. There were also chapters on integration of mental health into primary care, and effectiveness of traditional healers. Each chapter includes evidence from African researchers and guidelines for care. We used material available open access on the Internet to develop textbooks affording live links and a series of questions, which guided the students' reading of the research. While I was still in Rwanda, I met with faculty members and with the nurse in the Ministry of Health for feedback and guidance on the manuscript. We worked collaboratively so as to shape the textbooks appropriately for their use. There remain a few editorial issues that need to be resolved and then the manuscripts will be returned to Rwanda to be evaluated and hopefully utilized.

EPILOGUE

Many scholars have debated the African dilemma, asking, is it centuries of malnutrition that have disabled these proud people? Was it the slave trade that depopulated the continent, causing chaos and fear? Is it the political manipulation of despotic leaders that have crippled the economy? Or is it the continuing civil war that prevents people from having access to their land, and the peace of mind that comes from being self-sufficient? Or is it all of these historical tragedies that contribute to their continuing struggle today? I cannot answer this question and can only marvel at the resilient spirit that rises from the people—with whom I interacted—to begin each day joyfully.

I have to recognize that change comes very slowly. People tend to cling to the present moment and relish what they have. While they say that they want to learn, to improve, to change, the barriers are numerous and will require a collective will to overcome. They cannot simply speak it into being. It is only when some of the questions above have been answered and the issues have been resolved that words and reality will mesh and people can look to the future with the confidence that is required for sustained change to occur. For me to have been there, to have worked together with them, to have looked into their eyes, and heard the stories of genocide and recovery was transformational. The change in my life has been monumental.

12

Entre las Estrellas

Among the Stars

JANA MERVINE

Editor's Note: I was introduced to Jana Mervine by one of my students for whom she served as a preceptor in the global health course that I teach. Jana has a passion for travel and, like others represented in this collection, for sharing her nursing skills with the most vulnerable in the world. Jana identified a very creative strategy to support her avocation by becoming a travel nurse, an idea that I have shared with students. Through Entre las Estrellas, the nonprofit organization that she founded, Jana demonstrates that a small project can be a catalyst for change.

When I was 14 I had an opportunity to travel to Costa Rica with a mission group. I was introduced to "slums" for the first time. I had never seen people huddled under cars before, covered by cardboard boxes, sheltered by plastic and panhandling newspapers. Raw sewage was running down the streets as happy children, naive to their condition, played carelessly in the filth. For me, this begged the question: How can these children be so happy with so little, while at home, people are unhappy and have so much? It was an important realization for me, as it is for many people who witness joy coming from such unlikely places. My exposure to this extreme poverty shaped my worldview and changed the course of my life. That early spark of compassion grew into a burning desire to study something in college that could be used to make a difference in this world.

TEEN MANIA LEADS ME TO NURSING

I spent several summers in other countries working with Teen Mania. Teen Mania is a faith-based organization out of Texas that takes teenagers to underprivileged areas—giving teenagers an experience they are unable to have within the States. Teen Mania takes thousands of teenagers on 1-week to 2-month–long mission trips. These trips opened my eyes to what the world is made of. I was awestruck by the poverty and the conditions of so many people. After day one I was ready to commit my life to doing all that I could to educate these people and to give them other opportunities in life. Each trip provided more insight into what I would do with my life. It was where I learned that there are people in this world who can always benefit from whatever I am willing to offer.

I began my journey to make a difference in the world as a premed student in Indiana. However, this dream represented years of schooling and lots of debt. To expedite my plans to help the world, I changed my major to nursing. I felt that nursing would give me the ability to take a hands-on approach in helping the needy in the United States and abroad, without racking up insurmountable debt and over a decade of schooling. Nursing provided just enough challenges and opportunities to keep me interested, while the possibility of travel nursing confirmed my interest in the profession.

It seemed as if all of my interests and desires were aligning to lay the foundation to reach my goal. I chose to get my first bachelor's degree in Intercultural Studies and continued with an expedited 1-year bachelor of science in nursing in Miami, Florida. I packed my life into my car and drove from the doldrums of northern Indiana, to the tropics of the south Florida coast. When I arrived in a place where I had no friends or family, I was sure that I had made a mistake. This unfamiliarity would become routine for me. I persevered as I spent 7 days a week studying and doing clinicals, determined to learn everything that I needed to do to become a nurse.

ENROUTE TO TRAVEL NURSING

After passing the NCLEX, I had to spend a year gaining nursing experience in order to become a travel nurse. I decided that the excitement of the Trauma Intensive Care Unit fit my desire for adventure perfectly, but God had other plans for me. I ended up being hired in the Pediatric Emergency Room at the county hospital in Miami, a job I would never have predicted. I had always dreaded my pediatric clinicals and classes and had never even considered it as a specialty. Despite my initial opposition, 8 years later, I am still working in the Pediatric Emergency Room.

Following a painstaking year at an understaffed county hospital, where I had too many very sick patients and not enough resources to take care of them, I was finally able to refocus on my dreams. Travel nursing gave me the opportunity to work for an agency that helped me find a place to live and covered moving expenses. This satisfied my desire for adventure while easing my anxiety regarding the logistics of moving every 3 months.

My first travel assignment was in Philadelphia, where things were very different from the county hospital in Miami. I chose Pennsylvania because it was closer to home than I had been in many years, and the Children's Hospital of Philadelphia (CHOP) competes with Boston Children's for the number one children's hospital in the nation. I was forced to learn the CHOP way of doing things, leaving my "primitive" county hospital ways behind. The first 13 weeks were some of the hardest of my career. I was anxiety ridden every single shift, knowing that someone was going to point out something that I had done wrong. Someone was always looking over my shoulder to be sure that the new nurse was doing things their way. But, after much torture, I decided to extend my contract and to make the next contract a great learning experience. That is what I did. I picked up as many extra shifts as I could and made all the friends I could, and as a result became a much stronger nurse.

I continued to travel for 5 years. I had the opportunity to work in some of the best children's hospitals in the United States, including Rady Children's, Oakland Children's, Miami Children's, and Phoenix Children's. During my travels, I met and learned from some of the best nurses in the country. These hospitals, the nurses, doctors, and other staff, taught me things that I could never have learned otherwise. The things I learned would end up helping me in my profession long after, especially during my time in Ecuador. I also had the opportunity to work with nurses from all parts of the globe who gave me insight into nursing in places where I have never worked. I learned something from each and every one of those people.

Moving, changing jobs, new cities, new people, packing, and unpacking, has caused me to be more flexible both in my personal life and professional life. I can work with anyone, sleep anywhere, and be happy regardless of the situation. But what really satisfies me is my humanitarian work outside of my home country. Between travel assignments, I spent my time and money traveling.

SEEKING ADVENTURE

My preferred method is backpacking. This way, I get to experience the people and be immersed in the culture. During my travels all over the world, I fell in love with South America. I was consumed by the culture and developed an overwhelming desire to learn Spanish. I spent nearly 4 months traveling through a majority of the countries in South America. I was free to do anything on a whim. Because of this, I was able to do many things that only a handful of people have the opportunity to do.

For example, I have been in a prison in Bolivia where there is no security inside, only the inmates themselves who police the truly bad people. This prison is known for the quantity and quality of cocaine that inmates produce. It is also one of the few prisons in the world where the families of the inmates (spouses and children) live within the prison walls. I have traveled by bus into Colombia where they advised people like me not to travel because of the guerillas. I have been inside silver mines where men live very short lives because of the inhalation of toxic chemicals and the lack of oxygen. I have held a mother's hand in Haiti as her child dies of sepsis. I have held orphans in all parts of the world that only want someone to love them. Nothing else matters to these kids. They just want to have someone who will love them unconditionally. I have been handed a child in India by her mother and asked to please take her, to give her a better life in the United States. The love that it takes for a mother to do that is inspiring and saddening at the same time.

My travels have taken me beyond South America to Africa, Asia, Europe, and even road-tripping across North America. I have traveled in packed buses, strangers' cars, sleeper trains, boats in various states of disrepair, and large and small airplanes to get to wherever the wind is taking me. I have slept in hostels, on church floors, in convents, on beaches, and in strangers' homes. I have eaten mysterious meats, drank cloudy water, and snacked on strange creatures. I have survived parasites, bed bugs, and crossing some of the most dangerous boarders in the world. Along the way, I have met some of the most amazing people in this world. Life has given me millions of opportunities and I have taken every single one that has been given to me.

HAITI

In response to the 2010 earthquake in Haiti, I was invited to do relief work with University of Miami's Medishare and Samaritans

Purse. I seized the opportunity and ended up staying longer than I anticipated. While in Haiti, I experienced more sickness, suffering, and death than anyone should have to experience in an entire lifetime. Everyone seemed to be a victim of nature, violence, poverty, and/or disease. There was so much devastation and so much need. I knew this was where I needed to be; where my heart was gently tugging me.

On my first journey to this country, I volunteered with Medishare. They had set up a tent hospital at the end of the runway in Port-au-Prince. Devastating problems ran rampant as a result of the earthquake. There were burns, orthopedic injuries, sepsis, typhoid, malaria, and so many other disease processes with so little resources. Children were dying daily. There were only two or three nurses to care for 60 children. Working under those circumstances was one of the most trying times of my career as a nurse and in my personal life.

I met a young girl that I will never forget. Her family practiced voodoo and intentionally threw her into a fire because she had epilepsy—burning her from head to toe. By the time she arrived at the hospital, a few days later, she was pain ridden and gangrenous. She lay on the stretcher and stared, silent, in a catatonic state. When asked if she was in pain, no words left her mouth. We knew she was in pain, but realized she was more psychologically scarred than physically and was unable to do more than stare. We tried to manage her pain with medication, but her face revealed her true suffering. That is an image I will never forget.

I returned twice more to Haiti, once with Samaritans Purse and the next with Materials Management Relief Corp (MMRC). With Samaritans Purse, we went out into the community to set up a clinic for the day. People lined up for hours before we arrived. We saw every crippling disease you can possibly imagine. One case in particular involved a woman who was in her 90s and came to be treated for her headaches. She was in supraventricular tachycardia (SVT), or, a rapid heart rate. She could have been living with this heart rhythm for years. We tried everything to break it, but unfortunately we failed. She left in the same condition she arrived in. Another woman, who looked as if she was carrying a baby at full term, came to us lamenting that she had been pregnant for 2 years but had never felt the baby move and had yet to give birth. She had a tumor. She was sent to the Medishare hospital for treatment.

While with MMRC, I spent much more time in the streets of Haiti, living in a house where the rats and geckos ran freely. I slept on the porch where those varmints, I'm sure, came awfully close to me at night. But at least I could feel a slight breeze if there was one. During the day I worked at an HIV clinic set up in tents outside the hospital. I was with a doctor who had given up her career in the States to work in Haiti. Other times I had the privilege of working inside the hospital, taking care of children with seizures, sepsis, hydrocephalus, or physical injuries. We would also pick people up from wherever they lay to give them life-saving treatment.

Both organizations gave me an opportunity to work with suffering people. Their desperation in contrast with the awesomeness of their singing voices, when hope seemed lost, was inspiring.

Haiti held a special place in my heart, and I left with plans to return. However, shortly before doing so, a friend and fellow aid volunteer was wrongly imprisoned. He was accused of causing the death of a child. He had been working in the make-shift hospital, days after the earthquake, when a father brought in his septic son. The child died soon after arrival to the facility. Although my friend was at the hospital, he was a nonmedical volunteer and did not directly care for the child. We don't know what caused the father to single him out but, in any case, when his son died, the father accused my friend of wrong doing. To complicate matters, the father was unable to take the boy's body home, so it was cremated without his knowledge, which led to further misunderstanding.

My friend was imprisoned for 18 days in one of the most notorious prisons in the world. He was deprived of basic necessities. Food, clothing, and other items were provided by friends, as they advocated for his well-being while also trying every possible avenue for securing his release. He was eventually released and allowed to return to the States. After this incident, I was encouraged by him and others in Haiti to give it some time before I returned.

NEXT STOP: PERU

I was ready to continue working outside the United States on a more permanent basis, and Haiti gave me the courage to do so. It was what my heart had been telling me to do since my first trip at age 14. Although I couldn't go back to Haiti, I was determined to find another place where I was needed. Maybe not in the same way, but somewhere I could still make a difference. I was looking for an organization where I could volunteer without having a set structure or paying ungodly amounts of money to volunteer. I felt the pull of South America again. I would finally have an opportunity to learn to speak Spanish.

My adventure in South America started with an opportunity to work with Solidarity in Action. Solidarity in Action is a Canadian organization that takes college students to Peru and Ecuador to do community work. Through them I was given the opportunity to provide health assessments of school-age children. In Lima, there is a shortage of doctors. Because of this shortage, there are not enough people to check each and every child. I was sent to schools, orphanages, and daycares. In one of the orphanages, I treated kids covered in lice and scabies. My compassion for orphans consumes my heart. During these visits I met Clara.

Clara started an orphanage just by inviting street children into her home to learn to read. She now has about 50 children living in her home, where she tries to provide everything they need. She was a teacher in Lima for many years and noticed a lot of children near her home who were always in the streets. She began to invite them in and then could not send them back to the streets to sleep, thereby starting her orphanage. Now people from all over the world sponsor her project and help her to care for these children who are in need of so much. I miss Clara and the other 50 kids who touched my heart.

Lima has a large population of sick persons and not enough doctors to tend to them. This situation is particularly detrimental for underprivileged children in the area. Part of my job was to help the city of Lima create a database of specific issues that affect the poor. So in addition to checking for lice and treating scabies, I spent my days in elementary schools recording the heights and weights of the children. My limited ability to communicate in Spanish was frustrating. I went back to my humble accommodations each night with a headache. I was motivated to learn the language so that I could understand the children's stories—what they go through day to day. I wanted to know their dreams and listen to their thoughts about growing up. This experience made me realize that my ultimate dream is to start an orphanage.

FINDING A NICHE IN ECUADOR

Through contacts I made in Haiti, I was invited to help with a surgery program in southern Ecuador. We organized surgical teams to provide operations for people who otherwise do not have access to the care they need. In doing so, I met a man who invited a friend and I to a little mountain town in northern Ecuador. He showed us pictures and told us stories about Paragachi, and in no time we were on our way. Paragachi is where I fell in love with the people, the land, and the culture. It is now the place I call home.

Having worked with several nongovernmental organizations (NGOs), I realized that many of them require their volunteers to pay ridiculous sums of money to volunteer. However, that money may not directly benefit the people. It only took a few months of living in Paragachi and working with and researching organizations willing to help in my endeavors to decide that I wanted to start my own nonprofit. The result is Among the Stars/*Entre las Estrellas*, which began with the goal of putting every donated penny directly toward the betterment of the people it serves.

Starting a nonprofit in the United States is surprisingly simple. I printed the paperwork and completed it as instructed. I had a few people look it over and then submitted it. Apparently the recommended process is to consult with an experienced lawyer so that the forms meet government requirements. That was not an option since I was starting with limited funds. Fortunately, after making a few small changes Among the Stars Inc. was granted 501(c)3 status in the United States. *Entre las Estrellas* will soon be a legally recognized foundation in Ecuador, as well.

I currently work about 9 months of the year with *Entre las Estrellas* in Ecuador and spend the remainder of the year working to finance my avocation. I am committed to not using any donated money to finance my own expenses. I allocate all resources to benefit the people of Paragachi. These families have become my heart and my life.

Volunteers are invited for specific projects according to their background and their goals. Donations of items such as clothing and school supplies are accepted and financial donations are used for completing projects within the community. The purpose of *Entre las Estrellas* is to give people who live in this small Andean community the opportunities they deserve. Families or individuals in need of medical care are identified by our organization or are brought to our attention by others in the community. In addition to linking people with medical resources, we work with the entire family to provide assistance such as computer classes (computers were donated and sent to Ecuador), art classes in cooperation with another organization, and community education. We are dynamic. Once a need is identified, we collaborate with other organizations and the government to find resources to better the lives of these families.

We have assisted many children and families—for example, a little girl who was severely malnourished. She was brought to my attention by the day care, telling me that she could only eat pureed food and could not sit on her own. She only lay on her back, crying a weak cry. She was close to 2 years old and had not met any of her developmental milestones. I talked to the parents who agreed to have her seen, although in their opinion she was healthy and, like their previous four children, was just small. In the hospital, we ran genetic and other basic tests including a cat scan, which revealed that the brain had shrunken inside the skull. This poor child was suffering from nothing more than malnourishment. The mother had been feeding her only a cereal formula, which prevented her body from growing. After a diagnosis was made, she was treated with high-calorie formula, full-fat milk, and a diet to ensure she was eating every 3 hours without fail. With our intervention she has grown both in weight and length and is meeting her milestones! After treating this little girl, I was able to help the family with basic needs. A dentist in town offered to clean and fix the teeth of the entire family. The family was touched by simple things that those of us in the United States take for granted every day.

A 9-month-old child was brought to my attention because she was born with a flesh-colored hemangioma on the left temple; it had grown exponentially since birth. The mother had taken her to Quito to see specialists but was put on a waiting list for an injection that had to be ordered from China. Not only did the medication have to be ordered from China, there had to be at least four other children who needed it in order to make the process cost effective. After much persuasion, the injection was ordered for this individual child. She was treated. Her hemangioma has shrunken and she is growing and meeting all of her milestones.

MOTIVATION

Global work is rewarding! Small projects make huge changes! My life goal is to give people the resources they need to become successful! My motivation for doing global work comes from the attitude of the people. From my very first experience abroad, I knew that global work was my destiny. I was young, but I knew that I wanted to study something that would allow for me to travel, work, and make an impact on the world in some way. Health care seemed like a perfect opportunity. It gave me an avenue to not only give to people emotionally and physically, but to have a reason to begin a relationship with them as well.

My work as a nurse in the States and my work abroad has been an irreplaceable experience. I have chosen to dedicate my life to global work, but I encourage everyone, young or old, to experience the difference that they are capable of making in the world. The people we encounter are more than appreciative of every small gesture. From my early experiences in the slums of Costa Rica to my current life in Ecuador, I have learned more than I could have ever imagined about global work and my career in nursing.

There are many ways for people to participate in global work. My organization allows people to give with confidence that their hard earned money is not going to anyone's salary. All donors are given the option to give to a specific project, individual, or need. Whether it is a medical treatment for a specific child, transportation for volunteers, or to help bring a new educational program to the community of Paragachi, that is where your funds will go.

With the proper resources, there is no limit to the changes we can make in people's lives. There are always children who need to pay for school supplies, elderly to be clothed and fed, youth to be educated on health and hygiene, communities longing for social activities, or housing for a family in need. Among the Stars/*Entre Las Estrellas* is not bound by borders. We will not stop in Paragachi. Paragachi is only the beginning.

13

With Promises to Keep

Building Partnerships to Make a Difference

JENNY HARTSELL

Editor's Note: I've known Jenny Hartsell for several years in her role as preceptor for students enrolled in my global health course. Like Jana Mervine (Chapter 12), Jenny propelled her desire to serve onto a higher level by forming not just one, but two, not-for-profit organizations to support her global health endeavors. Jenny provides very practical advice for anyone wanting to establish their own nonprofit as she stresses the importance of communication and inclusion for establishing sustainable partnerships.

A bedpan bouquet of magnolias was waiting for me the day I graduated from nursing school in June of 1983. This gift, from my proud father, is a representation of where I am from and where my life has taken me. I grew up in Concord, North Carolina, a mill town of 35,000 people. Our family was middle class. My father had his own business; my mother was his secretary. Memories of my grandmother resonate fondly. She was funny, a little demented, and always full of stories. When her youngest son (my uncle) died, I was 15 years old. I flew to Florida with my grandmother and her children for the funeral. During the trip, I helped take care of her. She was an amputee with diabetes. That experience shaped my future. I knew, from that point on, that I wanted to be a nurse.

I started college as an education major, even though throughout high school I was in health occupations and wanted to be a nurse. What prompted me to change my mind when filling out my college application, I have no idea. It only lasted one semester. Several years later, I went back to study nursing and received my diploma from Cabarrus Memorial Hospital School of Nursing. That was more than 30 years ago.

Fast-forward 16 years to the year 2000, when I'm married to an emergency medicine physician, live in Texas, have two children, and too many animals. I quit my oncology nursing job 6 years earlier and had been volunteering and working on a bachelor's of arts (BA) in art part-time. My husband and I built and moved into our dream home.

At the insistence of a friend, I participated in a medical mission to Guatemala with a Baptist church group. I didn't want to go. I remember being terrified of leaving my safe life at home for a third-world country. Honestly, I had no point of reference for this type of work. No one I knew was in the Peace Corps. Growing up, we were taught that missionaries are saintly people and I was certain that was not me. My friend insisted that this work had my name written all over it. She was right. In the end, that week profoundly changed my life.

NONPROFIT BEGINNING

On that first trip to Guatemala, my friend and I worked in a rural hospital that was used only 1 week per year and was maintained by a governing board of 12 townspeople. Our team of about 50 volunteers included mostly laypeople plus a few doctors, surgeons, nurses, and interpreters. Our goal was to run simultaneous medical and surgical clinics. The first day, patients lined up and down the dirt street. One woman walked 70 miles and planned to walk back home after her surgery. There were families with small children camped outside the facility with little to eat. We worked 12-plus-hour days, had no running water, and slept in large bunkrooms with 30 other people. I barely slept, not from fear, but from excitement.

Returning home caused a distressing jolt to my reality. I remember not being able to buy clothing, struggling to buy anything but necessities at the grocery store, and questioning just about everything in my life. How could I live like I do, never wanting for anything, when so many people didn't have sufficient food, clean water, or basic medical care?

The next year, my friend and I decided to start a nonprofit to support travel twice per year to the same location, offering the community more frequent medical coverage. Our dream was for this hospital to become a year-round facility operated by Guatemalans with surgical teams coming in throughout the year. We dived in headfirst with no business or nonprofit experience and with a loose plan. Our hearts were in the right place, but we really did not know what we were doing. Looking back, I wonder if I would have taken the plunge, if I knew how challenging it would be. But what I now know is that my brave friend and some force beyond me provided the strength I needed to take a leap.

When I say we had no experience, I mean *zero* experience. During our first meeting, we adopted bylaws borrowed from the Klingon society, elected a fresh-out-of-college treasurer who bounced our very first check, and hired a lawyer who filed our organization with the IRS as a *for*-profit entity. Those weren't even our biggest problems. We needed money! On our first trip to Guatemala, we had traveled with a church group. They had an abundance of supplies, medications, and money. Churches have members. In the nonprofit world, they are called donors. This may seem like a nonissue, but nonprofits need public support to survive. Where were we going to get that kind of support? Neither my friend nor I liked asking others for anything; we just did everything ourselves. Not this time.

The first time we sent a letter asking everyone on our Christmas card list for money was painful. Our amazing friends and family generously gave their time and money, but truthfully, it wasn't enough. We had to be creative in finding money to support our new cause. Twice per year, we held auction fundraisers after going through our homes for antiques, gently used items, and emptying our jewelry boxes. Through trial and error, we realized passion is simply not enough. Starting and maintaining a nonprofit is a business, so we got to work reading, taking classes, and talking to people who were in the same business.

MOTIVATIONS AND EARLY LESSONS

Initially, my motivations were numerous but basically boiled down to one thing: I wanted to make a difference. I didn't speak Spanish, knew nothing about travel in Guatemala, and even less about the people, but I knew I needed to do something. The country's overwhelming need coupled with my need to help others became a marriage. Many people are wed to their jobs; I became wed to my volunteer job. At first, we struggled like any other couple. Some days were filled with bliss while others were filled with anger and sorrow, but most days were overflowing with contentment.

Early on, I was naïve, never asking myself enough questions, especially, "What will happen if I do blank?" Are there really consequences to helping people? One of my first big mistakes, believe it or not, was buying people gifts. The first few trips, I came bearing rewards to the local people who helped in the clinic. They were so grateful. It made me feel good to share with those who were serving their community. After a few times, the gifts became expected; requests were made, followed by requests for money. This might seem harmless, but what you don't realize at the time is that you are setting precedence. I had created a monster, and to my surprise, I began resenting that monster. I had to ask myself, "Is this what you've come to do?" It was so hard to take it all back once I went down that road. I guess I could've saved myself some anguish by setting some personal guidelines, "thinking before acting" being the number one rule.

Then there were those people I met on my travels, missionaries and local people who seemed to benefit significantly from others' misfortunes. Don't get me wrong, not everyone had his or her hand out. Ninety-nine point nine percent of the people I have encountered are lovely, warm, and hardworking. But, that small percentage of people who appear to be involved in helping others for personal gain makes you a little skeptical. I was devastated to learn there were people who were serving others out of self-interest. It took me a while to get past the disappointment. Staying connected to the people who were there to help was my salvation. I always reminded myself why I was there: to create an environment where people felt safe and cared for, a place where their basic health needs could be met.

For the next few years, my friend and I led medical teams of up to 60 volunteers twice a year to that same rural hospital, providing general medical clinics and surgery. The project was going well, but the community only had medical coverage 3 weeks per year: 2 weeks from our team and 1 from the church. What the area really needed was a full-time clinic and hospital. Could we be there all the time? Or, the better question: *Should* we be there all the time? With these questions in mind, my friend and I met with the 12 community members who supervise the projects to discuss the future of the hospital. The unanimous conclusion to the meeting was to make the dream of full-time service a reality. The local group tasked themselves with writing up the initial plan. We waited patiently.

After the first year, in addition to the 2 weeks of clinic in the Guatemalan countryside, we started taking small teams to another more isolated area of Guatemala twice per year. For 4 weeks out of the year I was in Guatemala running the medical clinics. During the rest of the year I was using skills I didn't know I had: marketing, fundraising, administrative, and organizational, among others.

Innovation and duct tape soon became my best friends. When you are in remote areas of a foreign country, you don't usually have modern conveniences or even what you truly need. Any round tube becomes a spacer for an inhaler, sticks become splints, and clothing a sling. This was when I realized my dad's gift—the bedpan of magnolias—had become my reality. When the flowers didn't have a vase, I found a solution to the problem. I was learning to think outside the box.

NEXT PHASE

After 3 years, I decided to leave the first nonprofit I helped conceive. This was one of the most difficult decisions I have ever made. For me, it was like giving up a child. But the truth of the matter is I could no longer stay engaged. This wasn't what I wanted to be doing. Our organization was helping thousands of people every year, but I felt pulled in a hundred different directions. I personally lacked focus, and at that time I couldn't honestly put my finger on what made sense for me. So, I stepped away. My friend continued on with the organization. In fact, that organization is strong and functioning in Guatemala today.

My next nonprofit adventure began because of a seating arrangement on an airplane. On my last trip home after working with the first nonprofit, my husband and I sat beside a U.S. Embassy employee whose wife volunteered for Safe Passage (Camino Seguro in Spanish), a project working with children living around the Guatemala City dump. His story of a courageous young woman from the United States, who dropped everything to bring education to impoverished children, was riveting. Over the next year, I corresponded with Safe Passage and visited the project with friends. In January 2006, physicians Marie Berkenkamp and Wright Hartsell, a dentist, Jeff Beal, and I created Shared Beat to help support education through health.

Our initial trips to this area were mostly fact finding. Our doctors provided annual physical exams to the 500 students in the Safe Passage educational reinforcement project, and we held biannual community clinics, opening the doors of the school to the neighborhood surrounding the dump. What an education this was for us! We had all worked in rural Guatemala, but Guatemala City introduced a whole new layer of complexity, especially regarding health. When you get right down to it, people are people wherever you go. We all have the same basic needs: water, food, and shelter. But when you add cultural and environmental factors, suddenly you are behind the learning curve again.

The microcosm of the Guatemala City dump and the surrounding neighborhood is fascinating. The inhabitants are Guatemala City natives, people from the Guatemalan countryside, and other Central Americans hoping to find work. On one of my first trips to Safe Passage, we visited a cemetery overlooking the city dump. Thousands of vultures sat in wait above, while below, thousands of dump workers scavenged through garbage for food, household goods, and items to sell. Others lined up behind garbage trucks.

The dump workers are recyclers. They sell their collections of plastic, glass, cardboard, and other items to large buyers and companies. When the world economy is bad, business for the recyclers is worse. They collect and store their recycled items in their homes until the market recovers—that means garbage in their house. Their homes sit adjacent to hillsides layered in trash. Many are made of salvaged materials. It is not uncommon for families of 6 to 10 people to live in a 10′ by 10′ space with no running water, cook on an open fire, and sleep in one bed. The people living in the dump community are amazingly resilient. These people and their families are our patients.

Our main objective at Safe Passage was and still is to keep the children well so they can stay in school. Sound simple? It would be without so many overwhelming obstacles to good health. People are inadequately nourished, drink contaminated water, live in makeshift homes, sleep with several other family members in the same bed, and have no indoor plumbing. Their homes are filled with trash, they live literally on top of one another, and their neighborhood is one of the most dangerous in Guatemala. Substance abuse and violence are commonplace. In the countryside, children cling to their mothers and rarely cry. In the city, the children are tough. I don't know how else to say it. They have an edge that comes from living in a world where danger is around every corner. An infant is cared for by a 6-year-old sibling while mom is at work. An 8-year-old steps around people who have been huffing glue and dodges cars and buses on the way to school.

Over the course of the first year and a half, we came to the conclusion that if we were to have a real impact on the students' health, we needed to make a full commitment. The twice-per-year outreach clinics were fun and somewhat beneficial but really only served as a Band-Aid for the real problems. In the fall of 2007, Shared Beat became a partner in health with Safe Passage. The children were already receiving hot meals and snacks at the project. We added daily vitamins, parasite prevention twice annually as prescribed by the World Health Organization, supported the clinic with much-needed medications and supplies, provided physical exams and follows-ups, and started from there.

Staying focused in an area with such challenging needs is more difficult than you can imagine. You treat a patient's diarrhea only to find they drink contaminated water. You give patients lice shampoo or scabies cream, and they go back to an infested home with no real way to get rid of the problem. You give a parent medication for a child's illness and say, "Have them take this with food," but they have no food, no money, and no job. Once the realization sunk in that we couldn't fix all the problems, I started going through the stages of grief: denial, anger, bargaining, depression, and finally, acceptance. The moment when you come to terms with the fact that you are not a superhero is humbling and, most importantly, necessary. That precise moment when you get over yourself is when you can start the real work.

Coloring the world black and white might be boring, but things would definitely be easier. We could say, "Our job here is to take care of medical issues. Period. End of discussion." But, then you have a young boy who, while salvaging materials to sell, receives a crush injury to his hand. He's treated in a local hospital and ends up with both a terrible infection and a gangrenous finger. His hand no longer resembles a hand. My husband, an emergency medicine physician, tells the boy his finger needs to come off or he'll lose his arm. He agrees to the procedure and the amputation goes well. While explaining his discharge instructions on how to take the medication, where to get follow-up dressing changes, and not to work until his hand heals, he stops us. In Spanish he says, "This is not possible. My family won't be able to eat." So, you've saved his hand, possibly his arm, maybe his life, and he won't follow discharge instructions? Sound familiar? A patient not following instructions definitely isn't unique to this area; it's a global problem. So, what do you do? In the end, we had the boy come to the local nurse for dressing changes. To encourage him not to work and further damage his hand, she gave him a day's wages every day for 2 weeks. He followed instructions because we took care of his burden, his hand healed, and he was able to go back to work after 2 weeks. We have given patients money for food but not started a feeding program; we have provided money for shoes but not created a clothes closet. Because the problems of the impoverished are enormous on all levels, it is hard to not want to fix everything. Wouldn't it be great if we could? Making a plan and staying focused is important. To avoid spreading yourself too thin, you have to constantly ask yourself, "What is our mission?" However, it is also important to remember that there are always going to be some gray areas.

ALLOWING PEOPLE TO SAY "THANK YOU"

Our first medical outreach at Safe Passage was a mix between wonderment and frustration. Our group was accustomed to working hard and doing things for themselves without much fuss. That week, Safe Passage assigned two team leaders to look after us and make sure all our needs were met. We were grateful for the extra assistance since it was our first week. The first day, we walked in to find an 8' by 3' table covered in tinfoil and filled with breads, fruits, sweets, water, and coffee. How wonderful, we thought. Well, this table was right in the middle of a 15' by 10' waiting area where patients waited to be seen by the doctor—hungry patients who had no food at home. We were told, "This is for you. *Do not let the patients have any!*" This was one of the hardest things our group has had to endure. We were walking a thin line between disrespecting our host and taking care of starving patients. Before too long, the volunteers started sneaking the food into exam rooms and giving it to the patients. On the second day, I broached the subject of removing the table, and our hosts were mortified that we didn't like their offerings. As volunteers continued to complain about the table and having to watch patients stare longingly at the food, I asked for the table to be removed, yet again, and replaced it with a smaller one offering coffee and water. As it turns out, I completely embarrassed and offended our host.

At the end of the week, the school shut down our clinic before we were finished seeing patients so the staff could have a goodbye party for our group. This seemed odd—we were only there for 1 week. There was cake, punch, group after group of speeches, and entertainment. It was very sweet and took a lot of time and effort to prepare, but we were embarrassed. Our goal for the week had been to assess and care for the sick and injured. A thank-you card made by some of the children would have been nice, but the food and goodbye party were excessive. The money spent on us could have been spent on the children. Yet what the staff was trying to do was show gratitude, and we essentially belittled their offering. Making the children feel better was all we needed, but undoubtedly we should have allowed them their traditions on this first trip and negotiated a lesser celebration of "us" the next time. Over the years, I came to realize that they thought we expected to be celebrated. When we came to an agreement that we didn't need the food or celebrations, we all felt relieved.

INCLUSION

When helping others, you need to always remember to include them in the discussion and the work from the very beginning. On that first trip, I made the mistake of thinking that we should work autonomously and give our host nurse and physician a break. Instead it made them think we were arrogant, didn't respect their practice, and were trying to take over. Looking back, I don't blame them. First of all, you are on someone else's turf. You need them. They know the ins and outs of the area and can help you. Second, if you are trying to change habits to a "best practice" model, you need to involve the people on the ground or they will not buy in to whatever you are selling. Communication and inclusion in decision making are two of the most important things I learned from this trip. I know I've learned those things before, but somehow I lost perspective in this new place.

This reminds me of a funny story regarding inclusion and knowing your audience. My husband, an emergency medicine physician, found out that the local ambulance drivers and emergency crews had no formal training. So, on one trip to rural Guatemala, he and one of the technicians who worked in the emergency room decided to give these fellows a lecture on how to handle emergencies. Five crews showed up in uniform with various types of emergency vehicles ranging from a pick-up to a modern, slightly used ambulance from the states. Once the crews got together, the entire day of teaching was derailed. The crews took over and started talking about what their jobs entailed. Each showed off their vehicles, not one of which had any medical equipment, supplies, or medications except for the fancy ambulance with an empty oxygen tank. My husband and the tech were beside themselves at first but realized halfway through the day that a meet-and-greet was a better idea anyway. They had no real idea what the job of these emergency crews entailed or what they had to work with and couldn't have effectively prepared a class without their audience in mind.

PARTNERSHIPS

One critical element in creating program success in the nonprofit world, especially in foreign countries, is cooperative partners. The synergy created by two groups working together for the same cause is hard to produce by one group alone. For example, Safe Passage provides funds for the students to attend public schools, homework reinforcement, social work, and extracurricular activities and makes a hot meal and snack available every day. Shared Beat focuses on health and prevention, providing health education, daily vitamins, a school clinic with clinic staff, medication and supplies, vision support, and biannual medical outreach clinics for the community. Safe Passage focuses on the child's education and family needs while Shared Beat concentrates on health. We each raise our own funds, create our own policies, and collaborate when issues arise. Together, we are strong and working toward the same goal.

Partnering with nonprofits or established organizations can help unravel logistical mysteries, legal questions, and sensitive cultural issues. Logistics while working outside your own country can be a nightmare! Working together with other organizations and/or nonprofits from that area creates an easier avenue for you to provide services. For example, the organization can help you choose the right site to hold a clinic or the correct way to travel to a location. Time you might spend on finding out where to stay, how to travel, and where to buy essentials for your work is time saved for other important things. Something as simple as reliable transportation can make or break your experience.

Partnering also allows you or your organization to work under the umbrella of the other groups. The nonprofit or organization should be aware of government rules and regulations and can help you work within the law. If they don't know something, they can find out who to ask much faster than you would be able to find out. There's no one better to help with cultural issues than people who live in that area! Whether it is the United States or Guatemala, there are certain cultural norms you should practice while visiting. For instance, on one of our medical outreach trips, we were asked to host a medical clinic in an area that was supporting mudslide victims. Our medical team saw more than 100 patients that day, and as a thank-you, some of the ladies in the community cooked lunch for the group. As a rule, we always bring peanut butter sandwiches for everyone, but they insisted our team eat with them. What they served was gray, crinkled flesh swimming in tomato sauce. The group had to ask, "What is this called?"

Tripe, they said. We know it better as intestines. Everyone dug in and did the best they could to not embarrass our hosts. Of course, there was a little tripe left hiding under our napkins, but it was important to be respectful.

Shared Beat began as a nonprofit to support Safe Passage's goals. But over the past few years, we've also started working with rural nonprofits and education projects by providing year-round vitamins, parasite prevention, scholarships, and community clinics. We have found by working hand-in-hand with other nonprofits and educational programs that we are able to do more with our money. This concept has proven to be beneficial to all concerned, especially the people we serve.

MEDICATIONS AND SUPPLIES

When I first started working with nonprofits going to Guatemala, we obtained our medications through donations. Taking donations is wonderful if you can get large enough quantities to make a difference. However, if you are getting four sample capsules of an antibiotic, three sample tablets of a diuretic, and two samples of Viagra (I am not kidding), you not only don't have what you need, but you also have wasted extra time sorting, counting, and removing packaging from medications that you may not be able to use.

Over the years, we have developed a formulary of medications based on the illnesses and diseases we see frequently. We have identified nonprofits that support other nonprofits by providing quality, essential medications, and supplies at a fraction of the cost you would normally pay at a pharmacy or pharmacy supply. Blessings International in Broken Arrow, Oklahoma, has an extensive formulary of medications and supplies. For our vitamin needs, we either purchase from Blessings International or from Equipping the Saints in Weyers Cave, Virginia. Using one or two sources makes the process less complicated and time consuming. Over the past decade, most pharmaceutical companies have changed their policies and are now donating to organizations like MAP International, who also provide medications to nonprofits. MAP offers prepared packages of medications that could be exactly what you need to provide care. One word of caution: Don't take medications or other items that are out of date or damaged. Do not accept donations of nursing textbooks, for example, that are older than 5 years. In other words, do not donate items that would not be acceptable for use in the United States. To do so represents unsafe practice and is often perceived by the receiving organization as demeaning.

WHAT DOES NURSING HAVE TO DO WITH IT?

Over the past 13 years I have spent working in Guatemala, only a small percentage of my time has been devoted to actual hands-on nursing. I am a diploma nurse graduate. We trained for 3 years in hands-on nursing, getting to the root of problems and fixing them. After graduation, I became an oncology nurse. I loved it. Oncology encompasses every body system. There are the technical parts and other aspects like relationship building, listening skills, the ability to see gray, and the incredible strength required to help someone approaching the end of his or her life. My nursing education and career helped to prepare me for the diverse, physical, and emotional role of working in the global health environment. I am not saying that my experience in nursing before Guatemala completely prepared me, but I am able to draw on that time and apply it to the challenges of working with the impoverished in a foreign country.

The continual triage plus knowing the equipment, supplies, and medications make having a nurse in charge of medical outreach beneficial. Yet I have also been on medical outreach where laypeople were in charge, and it worked. Whoever is in charge needs to be motivated to make things function and prevent them from falling apart when they don't. Just because you have a nurse in charge doesn't mean things will go well. I have been on trips where a nurse was in charge and because of the lack of preparation before the trip and the lack of leadership during the trip things did not run smoothly. That doesn't mean do it all yourself. Delegate, but make sure to follow up. Remember: In most instances, this is a volunteer job.

Planning can be complicated, especially for the first trip, so don't be afraid or too proud to talk with other people who have done similar work. Collaborate and learn as much as you can from others. Trip planning includes preoutreach, outreach, and postoutreach. Preoutreach involves recruiting medical and ancillary volunteers, ordering medications and supplies, developing medical and volunteer forms for documentation, preparing schedules and logistics, communicating with your hosts, and learning as much as you can about the area. During the outreach, you are busy helping set up pharmacy and triage, taking blood pressures, checking blood sugar levels and teaching others how to do them, reading doctors' orders, making judgment calls on testing, disease and medication education, feeding volunteers, and keeping them safe. After the outreach, there are follow-up medical calls, data collection, entry, and reporting.

Over the years, I have led or helped lead more than 20 medical teams to Guatemala. I've worked with some amazing people, medical and nonmedical. Watching the nursing students perform blood sugar tests for the first time, seeing our vision team make a pair of glasses, and observing our doctors' gentle bedside manner motivate me beyond words. The camaraderie of volunteers working closely together for a week in a foreign land, sometimes for the first time, is like magic. Lifelong friendships are forged, career decisions are made, and most everyone's perspective changes a little. Some groups are more magical than others. Only on a few occasions have we had that one person who brings friction—the party pooper; the sophomoric volunteer who has never been on an outreach trip but on the first day has a better plan than your current one; or the volunteers who were expecting to work alongside Hawkeye Pierce in *M*A*S*H* before learning that instead they are helping with monotonous children's physical exams. It is not that they weren't told what they would be doing ahead of time. People may not admit it, but they do have an agenda when they sign up for these trips, and learning early on that you will not be able to please everyone saves an enormous amount of headache and heartache.

A few times throughout this great adventure, being a nurse was truly an advantage. Our group, Shared Beat, provides salary support, medications, and supplies for the clinic at Safe Passage. The clinic is operated by a professional Guatemalan nurse and a part-time Guatemalan doctor. From time to time, the nurse has been absent while I was visiting Guatemala. So, I have been able to substitute for her for a week here and there. Then, when the clinic lost the school nurse, during the search for a new one I substituted for 1 month. I'd like to share a few excerpts from my blog during that time.

JANUARY 2011

Arrival: I arrived back in Guatemala last Monday for 5 weeks — my longest trip of 30 to this country in more than 10 years. I have to say, I'm pretty excited. My enthusiasm is a result of my purpose. For the next 4 weeks, I will act as the school nurse in the Safe Passage school clinic. The last week, our medical team of 17 will be here, but until then, I'm on my own.

Guatemala always welcomes you with that noxious smell of diesel! It sounds a little crazy, but that familiar smell is as comforting to me as the smell of pound cake coming from my grandmother's kitchen. I know I'm back when that airplane door opens and it hits me in the face. What does that smell mean? Soon I'll be surrounded by the smiling faces of 500-plus children from the Guatemala City dump community. And hugs, millions of hugs! That smell feels like home.

Being a school nurse was an amazing yet frightening experience. The Safe Passage clinic acts as school clinic, quick care and emergency room all in one, seeing an average of 25 people per day, ages 0 to 80. It was one of the most gratifying and exhausting experiences of my life. I wouldn't trade it for anything!

First day: I saw lots of "boo boos," half the school had a stomach bug, and the other half had colds. Add in the children from daycare. It definitely takes a little extra patience and maybe a colorful sticker to finally win them over. Now, throw in their parents and community members. Pregnancy, hypertension, diabetes and burns . . . you get the picture. They have so much going on. Many of them work in the dump, are single parents, and live in makeshift homes with leaky roofs. Did I mention the employees? You have to make them better. They keep the place running. And let's not forget the volunteers! They are awesome, and most of them are thousands of miles from home. Many are in their late teens, away from home for the first time, in a foreign country, traveling, eating strange foods, and who knows what else! Do they have traveler's diarrhea? Could it be Malaria? There are so many things to consider in this community quilt.

Pint-size hypochondriacs: I saw more than 50 people in 6 hours and am having trouble thinking in English or Spanish. Every day, I am amazed at the resilience of the people who live here. Every day, there are things that make me a little sad and lots of things to make me laugh. For instance, did you know that hypochondriacs come in every size and from everywhere? This one child comes to the clinic almost every day. It's like watching a Saturday Night Live *skit each time she visits. I say, "What's the problem?" She says, "Um, well, I have pain in my elbow—yeah, my elbow." Then I ask if she hurts anywhere else, every part confirmed, even the eyelashes. Her medicine: a hug! My pay: a beautiful, snaggle-toothed smile.*

BEST PRACTICE: SUSTAINABILITY

Media plays a big role in medicine today. Just like remedies concocted and passed down through generations, no matter where you are in the world, it is hard to change someone's mind about what they believe is the best antidote to their problem, whether they heard it on TV or from grandma. This makes it difficult to develop "best practice" standards in medicine. In the United States, people go to their doctors and say,

"My neighbor said that I need antibiotics." In Guatemala, people can walk up to the pharmacy and spend their grocery money for the week on antibiotics without a prescription. The culture in regard to access to medication is hard to change. People want a quick fix to their problems, not unlike the United States, but Guatemalans can essentially practice medicine. At first, this was frustrating beyond reason. But what can you do? Being a foreigner doesn't help in most instances, and how can you compete with grandma's advice? You need trust and education.

Barreling in to save the world doesn't work except in disaster situations. If you want to bring lasting benefits to a community, best practice, and sustainability, you first have to establish trust—much like Hanley, the schoolteacher who started Safe Passage. She started her program by feeding children out of a church. The community grew to trust and love her and believed in her because she believed in them. Unfortunately, Hanley, the "angel of the dump," was killed in a car accident in 2007. What she started lives on today with more than 550 students in the program and has become a true model of sustainability. When I first started going to Guatemala, I remember making promises and being met with a "we will see" attitude. What I didn't understand at the time was that people come to places like Guatemala, are shocked by what they see, and have every intention of coming back. But they never do. If you promise, make good on your promise. Hanley made good on her promises, and people believed.

Once you establish trust, people are more likely to listen when you have something to say. Dispelling myths, correcting local doctors with questionable practices, and changing "known" facts takes time, education, and a gentle finesse. Nothing really says sustainability like education. We started one-on-one health education with the children during their physical exams. Next, we added the adults when they came to our outreach clinics. From time to time, we held educational classes for the students and adults. A few years later, a Safe Passage volunteer created a health education program and helped obtain a grant to get it started. After the grant expired, our group took over fiduciary responsibility. Now each child in the program receives 30 minutes of health education, mostly prevention, twice per month. The 50 or so adults in the adult literacy program receive health education once per week. Sharing even the smallest health secrets can have an enormous trickle-down effect. Nothing has given me greater pleasure than having an 8-year-old run up to show me how to cough appropriately or seeing children wash their hands correctly after going to the restroom. It really is the little things.

In 2009, Shared Beat established a scholarship program to provide resources for students who want to pursue a career in health care. The program was designed for traditional students in their late teens, but shortly after establishing our guidelines we were approached by an adult literacy teacher asking why we wouldn't give scholarships to the moms. Subsequently, our first two recipients were moms. We've had three women graduate as nurses, two as nursing assistants, and five who have graduated from preparatory classes in science. Providing resources for the students guarantees resources in the future for the community: nurses, nursing assistants, and one day, doctors. One of our main goals is to work ourselves out of a job!

REFLECTIONS

Working in Guatemala has changed my life. The rewards are numerous. Practicing in the same area and providing consistent preventative and basic care does change people's lives. When we compare the student population at Safe Passage to other student populations in Guatemala City and rural Guatemala, the difference is remarkable.

If you do decide to start your own nonprofit, make sure you have a good support system, get a hardworking board of directors, talk to others who have done similar work, and make a plan. Starting a nonprofit organization is much like having a baby. If you really considered all of the consequences, possible dangers, and pitfalls beforehand, let's be honest in saying most of us would opt to go childless. After starting two health care service nonprofits, I realize that I have few regrets. The pain turned into life lessons for me and, hopefully, a few changed lives. The experience continues to enrich my life every day, much like my children do.

I would like to leave you with two challenges. One, discover the part of yourself that, when faced without a vase, you would choose a bedpan. Two, take that leap, whatever it may be. Just don't forget your parachute!

14

Changing Lives for the Better

A Week With Shared Beat in Guatemala

JANE CALTHROP

Editor's Note: Jane Calthrop lived abroad as a child and drew upon those experiences to shape her goals for nursing. As a nursing student, she traveled with a medical team to Guatemala. Jane discusses important lessons she learned regarding motivation, flexibility, and resourcefulness. She shares her belief that, with teamwork exhibiting these attributes, short-term global experiences can have a positive impact on the nurse as well as the people she is serving. Jane met objectives for the global course Practicum in Nursing; Global Health Experience, mentioned in the Preface, through her volunteer work with Shared Beat. *Jenny Hartsell (Chapter 13) served as her preceptor for this experience.*

I am a nursing student at the University of North Carolina, Chapel Hill, tackling my third career! My first degree was in pharmacology, and I worked for many years in the pharmaceutical industry. Later I moved into Human Resources as an employee training and development specialist and went on to obtain a master's in education. However, after being laid off in 2006, I realized I needed to make more of a difference in the world and decided at the grand age of 48 that the time was right to become a nurse. My husband has a steady job with health benefits, so we decided we could afford to take the risk. I felt that this new career path would allow me to combine my love of sciences and health with my ability to work with people and build relationships in order to provide hands-on care and education to enable people to live healthier, longer lives.

MOTIVATION FOR GLOBAL WORK

During the summer after my junior year in nursing school, I had the opportunity to enroll in a global health course and to go abroad to expand my clinical experience. This greatly appealed to me as I grew up in several countries (Sri Lanka, Malaysia, Singapore, Zambia, and England) and love to travel and experience new cultures. My upbringing exposed me to the many inequities that exist around the world, fostering in me a deep compassion for those less fortunate than myself. These experiences were foundational to my development of a strong sense of justice and a need to contribute to efforts to help redress some of these inequities. As I grew up, I became acutely aware of my privileged childhood as a wealthy expatriate, and how lucky I was to be born into a family that was able to take advantage of the many opportunities available to us. As an adult, I have been a regular volunteer, sharing my time and experience with at risk kids, low-literacy adults, and victims of domestic violence. As a result, I feel a pull toward Public Health nursing, and realized that a clinical experience in another country would be valuable to me both professionally and personally. In addition, I wanted to improve my Spanish language skills, so I knew that a Central or South American country would be an ideal destination for this experience.

I signed up to volunteer for a week with a not-for-profit medical outreach organization called Shared Beat, based in Texas. Its mission is to "empower children and their families through health and wellness care and education so they can achieve self-reliance and a positive future." Their focus is Guatemala, where Shared Beat provides direct primary care for 1 week every 6 months to approximately 1,000 people in Guatemala City and several surrounding rural villages. They partner with other locally based, not-for-profit organizations, such as Camino Seguro (Safe Passage, in English), which runs a school for approximately 600 children of workers in the city dump, and Common Hope, which focuses on education, health care, and housing. Through these and other local connections, they maximize their impact by both enhancing their understanding of the cultural needs and increasing access to their target populations. The trust between Shared Beat and the local clients they serve is growing as they continue to provide a consistent and reliable service over the years. In addition, Shared Beat has established a permanent school clinic based at Camino Seguro and funds the salary of a full-time school nurse and a part-time physician. They also fund a number of scholarships to assist students in achieving a college education and professional qualification in the health care field.

MY ROLE

My role as a student nurse during my week with Shared Beat was to help out and learn as much as possible. There were 28 volunteers from the United States in the group: some medically trained, some students, some organizers, and several Spanish interpreters. We divided into groups and worked simultaneously in several locations each day. Each day the teams arrived early at their sites to set up the clinic and supplies, which included a large variety of medications, blood pressure cuffs and stethoscopes, glucometer kits, urinalysis strips, a scale, dressings, syringes, and bottles. Small private rooms or an area closed off with a sheet were used for client consultation by one of the providers—there were two pediatricians and one gastroenterologist—and benches were set up in the waiting area for clients. There was a check-in desk to admit the clients and provide them with a form that was to be completed throughout their visit. At Camino Seguro, there was a vision testing station and a room for physical therapy consultation. I took blood pressures, weighed the children, tested blood glucose levels, performed urinalyses, and worked closely with the person in charge of pharmacy to fill the medication orders and dispense the medications to waiting clients. I spent some time observing the physicians during consultations with the clients. The majority of clients were women and their children. In addition, I conducted some vision tests and was part of the fluoride team, providing toothbrushes and applying fluoride to the teeth of approximately 1,500 school children during the week. A number of the Shared Beat team members were "old-timers," having participated on these trips many times, and the rest of us were first timers, but hopefully not last timers! The days flew by as we were very busy trying to see as many patients as possible, and minimize the number we had to turn away. I had to get up to speed with the processes quickly, practice my newly acquired Spanish language skills, be attentive to the needs of the team and our clients, and be flexible and willing to help out where needed.

LIVED REALITY

The people we treated survive under very difficult circumstances. They lived in small, mud-floor houses, slept in close quarters on floor mats often with flea-ridden dogs and cats, cooked on internal wood-burning fires that are not vented to the outside, and lacked potable water, with a penchant for early-age consumption of locally grown coffee. Many of the city squatter communities had no running water, electricity, or proper sanitation, resulting in crowded and unhygienic conditions, leading to a number of diseases and conditions, such as parasitic worms, fleas, lice, scabies, dermatitis, diarrhea, and gastritis. Many men worked in physically demanding jobs such as farming and construction, and some of our clients work in the city dump, which is rife with toxic chemicals and physical hazards. Most women had many children and toted the baby around on their backs while cleaning and keeping house. The strenuous physical labor commonly results in back, neck, and other joint pains and types of injuries. The Shared Beat staff was well prepared to treat conditions common to rural and squatter life, including parasites, back pain, headaches, rhinitis, allergies, asthma, gastritis, diarrhea, eczema, and dermatitis. The urban population in Guatemala City experiences a higher prevalence of noncommunicable, chronic diseases such as diabetes, hypertension, hyperlipidemia, and obesity for which the team was prepared to treat with 6 months' supplies of relevant medications and health prevention information about diet and physical activity to tide them over until the next Shared Beat visit.

COLLABORATION

The most striking aspect of working with Shared Beat was the extraordinary sense of teamwork and collaboration I experienced amongst the team members. Even though it was often stressful working at a fast pace in order to see at least 100 patients per day at each location, we all worked really well together. I was delighted to find that we bypassed much of the "forming," "storming," and "norming" behaviors that new teams typically experience, jumping straight to "performing" at a high level. I believe this was due to the strong leadership, the clear mission and goals of the team, and the can-do, flexible attitudes of each member. We checked in with each other, willingly volunteered to help where needed, swapped roles to give others a break or different experiences, and commiserated with each other's aching feet, backs, heads, and so on. As a student, I appreciated everyone's patience with me as I got up to speed, and others' willingness to teach me, such as inviting me to listen to a patient's heart murmur. There is something special about a group of people who travel on their own time and money to impoverished places to do this kind of work. Their rewards are purely intrinsic—being part of a team that is contributing to others' needs, and sharing this common vision with other like-minded people. We'd share our snacks on the long bus journey back to the hotel, eat dinners together, and spend our evenings exploring Antigua. Sometimes we'd sit in the hotel's quiet, beautiful garden overlooking the Volcan de Agua, chatting about the day, and sharing our stories. There were three other nurses on the trip, all with a wealth of experience. They were all inclusive, and shared their experiences and suggestions about my path into nursing. They were very encouraging and helped confirm my new career direction. Many had stressful nursing jobs and I believe they saw this trip as a welcome break and a way to donate their expertise to a worthwhile cause in a beautiful part of the world. I feel privileged to have been part of such a passionate, smart, caring, and fun team, and enjoyed getting to know these amazing people. I have stayed in touch with some of the team members and perhaps may even work with them again on future trips.

LESSONS LEARNED

My experience in Guatemala helped me to grow as a person and as a future nurse. The trip reconfirmed for me that I really enjoy being part of a tightly knit, functional, and highly motivated team, intent on making a positive impact on others. I liked the fact that we were all working together with limited resources and space, having to be flexible and resourceful. Although we had specific roles, most people were flexible, as needed. No task was too small or menial for anyone to take on, no question too stupid to ask, no explanation too much trouble to give. We were all there for the patients and wanted to serve as many as possible each day. I like being busy, having a task to do, keeping up with demands, and helping the clients get through the process efficiently, while still having a moment to chat with clients or laugh with a team member. We were there because we had chosen to be there. I realize that I need to find this kind of work environment when I graduate—one where I'm part of a team of self-motivated, smart, dedicated, caring, and fun people who want to be there doing what they do best.

Another lesson I learned was that I would like to have been more proficient in Spanish before my trip. It was a struggle and often exhausting to learn so much in such a short time. I took French in high school so I had no foundation in Spanish, just some experience with the process of learning a language. I made a huge effort to learn and speak the language by living with a host family and taking Spanish classes the week prior to working with Shared Beat. This immersion forced me to listen and talk as much as possible, and I was grateful to my host family for their infinite patience as I practiced my newly acquired knowledge with them. I was impressed by the proficiency of many of the Shared Beat team members who spoke Spanish with the clients. I noticed the difference this made in developing rapport and building trust, which will naturally improve the quality of care provided. The presence of several interpreters was key to working with those of us with a limited grasp of the language. I also learned that just making an effort to speak the local language is usually appreciated. We communicate on so many levels, and much can be conveyed with a few words and our body language. Smiling and hugging are universal, it seems!

This experience will help me be more appreciative of cultural differences: to find out why things are done in certain ways and not make assumptions or judgments before understanding the reasons and typical practices. For instance, many school-age children had caries, missing, and crooked teeth. They thought nothing of their dental situation and had ready wide grins for us! I found it horrifying that such young children already had so many blackened, jagged, and missing teeth. How terrible, I thought. Why don't they look after their teeth? What are their parents doing? I learned that there is no fluoride in village water and many mothers do not have the tools or knowledge to care effectively for their children's teeth. Although there seems to be a general acceptance of the situation, it did provide an educational opportunity to, sensitively, help them learn how to care for their teeth. We applied fluoride, provided toothbrushes, and explained how to mix a solution of baking soda and water to use in lieu of toothpaste.

Another key insight was the first-hand close-up exposure to the terrible conditions that some people are born into, such as the squatter communities that surround the Guatemala City dump, and the isolation and marginalization experienced by indigenous people, many of whom live in remote rural villages. Few have access to quality health care or the ability to pay for quality services and medicines. In some cases, even basic services such as clean water, sanitation, and electricity are an unaffordable luxury. I can imagine how hard it must be to find ways to change circumstances without adequate resources.

I was distressed to learn about the huge economic divide between the rich and poor in Guatemala, which apparently has one of the worst economic disparities in the world. My home-stay exposed me to a middle class family who, while living a simple life by our standards, appeared to have the means, education, and motivation to make the best of their opportunities and live good, happy, and healthy lives. They were a tight-knit family that valued their relationships and were constantly helping and supporting each other in many ways. Then I saw the city dump and the surrounding squatter communities—the other end of the spectrum. My heart went out to these people—our clients—who were for the most part so friendly and appreciative of our services. I believe this experience will help me be more compassionate with my future patients, and think about the circumstances that have led to their current situation and health problems. Even if some problems appear to be self-inflicted (for example, smoking, drinking, poor diet, lack of exercise), there may be many reasons why this is so. These include a lack of education or knowledge to understand consequences or find alternatives; depression or lack of hope, which negatively impacts motivation; societal models, norms, and peer pressure; lack of funds; lack of time, and so on. This humbling experience with Shared Beat—a team that gives their heart and soul to helping the needy—makes me appreciate what I have, and how lucky I am, and how I will soon be in a position to help improve the lives of others less fortunate than me.

Finally, I learned that a clear vision and the hard work of a handful of people that make up Shared Beat's Board and the dedication of caring professionals who volunteer their time and skills once or twice a year can make such a difference. Not to change the world, nor to make large systemic changes, nor even impact a huge population, but to help a few people in need. It was heartwarming to see what can be done with a healthy dose of drive, determination, passion, and resourcefulness. This experience inspired me and I believe that someday I will do something just as wonderful—to help change a few people's lives for the better, whether back home in the United States, or anywhere in the world.

15

From Foot Soaks to Self-Care

A Nursing Response to Homelessness

MARGARET THORNTON

Editor's Note: Margaret Thornton (Peggy—to her friends) illustrates that global health and public health are two sides of the same coin and that "global really is local." Peggy writes with great compassion as she describes her many years of volunteer work with a program in Boston serving the homeless. Her discussion regarding the importance of honoring relationships resonates throughout many of the narratives in this series.

My family and peers helped bring me to a career in nursing and my mother was my role model. She had always wanted to be a nurse but completed high school at 16 and no nursing school would accept her at that age. Instead she worked in the business world until she married. Although six children were born in 8 years, she found time to help others: errands for a shut-in, rides for an elderly neighbor, and occasionally taking in and caring for sick relatives. Pictures of children taken from a mission magazine our parents subscribed to were posted on the refrigerator. We were encouraged to think of a world far from our own where poverty was a given.

When deciding on a career, the possibilities I considered were teaching and nursing. My best friend chose teaching and being around children appealed to me. Yet the more I processed my options with classmates and friends, the more I was drawn to nursing. Making a difference in the health of individuals seemed a most worthy calling.

My nursing education includes a 3-year diploma program, bachelor's of science in nursing (BSN) and master's of science in nursing (MSN) in community health nursing, and certification as an adult nurse practitioner. I moved to Boston in 1973 as a single mother with two school-age children and needed a daytime nursing position. After 3 years of medical/surgical nursing and 2 years of community health nursing, I accepted employment at the Boston TB Control Project.

PINE STREET INN

The highest incidence of tuberculosis (TB) was in the neighborhood known as the South End, where the Pine Street Inn Shelter for the homeless was located. I understood that a nurse had been assigned to the shelter from the TB project because of the high number of cases seen there. I visited the shelter as part of my orientation as a TB nurse. Many who stayed at the shelter came to the TB clinic for evaluation. These individuals were frequently noncompliant with appointments as well as medication regimes because of substance abuse and/or mental illness, resulting in repeated hospitalizations.

I had witnessed the impact of substance abuse (namely alcoholism) and mental illness in my own family as well as in those with whom I grew up: a grandfather needed to be coaxed home from the bar; an aunt was unable to tend to her young family; there was insufficient food in my childhood friend's home (a mayonnaise sandwich would be lunch) because her alcoholic father was not working. This behavior was whispered about and judged in unfavorable terms by adults I was close to. My view of substance abuse and mental illness as a youngster was therefore negative. Experience as a nurse changed my attitude: I learned to see these individuals as being ill and deserving of care much, as were people with heart disease.

I arrived at the shelter during orientation week somewhat nervous, never having been to a shelter before. It was housed in an old rambling warehouse-like building bordering Boston's Chinatown. Inquiring for the nurse, I found myself in a mammoth cave-like space, dark and smoky, occupied by men of all ages in shabby clothing and in various states of uncleanliness. They were sitting on benches, lying on the floor; some were walking in circles, mumbling to themselves.

The counselor answering the door appeared very much at ease with what seemed like chaos to me. He led me into an office and introduced me to Barbara McInnis, the TB nurse, who was to become a mentor and role model for the rest of my career. She had an open, no-nonsense manner and answered my questions patiently, pointing out the importance of *relationship* to effective help, and respectfully referred to all residing at the shelter as *"guests."* She suggested that I observe her interviewing a new guest with TB.

After receiving permission from the guest for me to be present, Barbara began by stressing the importance of taking medicine regularly, possible side effects of the medication, and the importance of keeping clinic appointments. Since the interviewee admitted to alcoholism, this issue was also addressed, and detox services were offered. Barbara then asked where he was from, how he had come to be at the shelter, and how he spent his day. This was not a typical nursing assessment. Barbara McInnis indeed demonstrated the importance of *relationship*, a key to achieving resolution of the guest's TB, which could perhaps lead to reclaiming his life. Barbara also told me about the nurses' clinic at the shelter.

NURSING CARE

By 1973, the clinic had been in place for 3 years when Paul Sullivan, director of Pine Street Inn, recognized the need for health services and approached staff at Boston City Hospital who knew the shelter guests best—the emergency room nurses. The nurses understood the consequences of fragmented care: return visits to the emergency room with even more complicated presentations because of unfilled prescriptions, unchanged dressings, or sutures left in too long. They agreed with Paul Sullivan that nursing interventions were appropriate for the needs of this population. During the first years of clinic operation, all care providers were nurses and *all* were volunteers. The goals formulated for the clinic and the Inn were survival and, eventually, self-care.

When Barbara told me that care was provided in the room where we were sitting, I looked around at the tight quarters and thought, how is this possible? As if reading my mind, she responded: "Oh, we clear our director's desk next door and use it for an exam table." A quick glance revealed an area no larger than the one we were in. A closet-sized bathroom was the sole private space, and that was the extent of "the clinic!"

As I was leaving, a guest experienced a seizure. An impeccably dressed man in a suit and tie knelt down on the floor next to the guest and assisted us in turning him on his side. The well-dressed man reassured the guest after he woke while Barbara called an ambulance. I asked her about the man who was helping us. It was Paul Sullivan, Pine Street's director. This was indeed an unusual place—caring people attending to broken people—in a clinic with nurses at the helm! My 27-year affiliation with the shelter began soon after that incident: I had decided to volunteer in the nurses' clinic.

I arrived at the shelter as a new volunteer with excitement and looking forward to the experience. Barbara was there to continue my orientation. Nurses were primary care providers here and *a nursing model was followed for delivering care*, with emphasis on an individual's response to health and illness. The guest was allowed to decide what his needs were but consideration of substance abuse and mental illness by caregivers was necessary, given the high incidence of both conditions at the shelter and the impaired judgment that so often accompany them.

While reviewing the clinic manual, I learned that the format or categorization was not based on a medical model (organized according to disease) but, rather, based on a response to a condition. Nursing provided the context; for example, *interference with thought processes*, *life style*, or *coping mechanisms* in contrast to *depression*, *anxiety*, or *schizophrenia*. Protocols were developed for the more common presentations such as malnutrition, risk of falls, and exposure to heat and cold.

RELATIONSHIP-BUILDING

I noticed that as guests lined up at the clinic door, lay volunteers wrote down names and requests in a log. Needs ranged from vitamins to referrals for detox. Foot soaks were popular and provided a strong link to the value and practice of relationship-building that Barbara had emphasized during our first meeting. Guests didn't seem to mind the crowded conditions and chatted amicably with staff and other guests as they soaked their feet; the many hours of walking the streets took a heavy toll on their only mode of transportation. Foot soaks thus became an integral part of the caregiving and relationship-building process. I could also see how this nurturing and accepting environment prompted the men to identify other health issues that may otherwise have gone unattended.

There certainly were the expected tasks—first aid, changing dressings, and taking vital signs, but nurse volunteers had other duties as well. These included triaging guests as they presented at the clinic; making rounds in the lobby of the building and its alley; conferring with counselors concerned about a guest who had failed to keep an appointment at the clinic; writing referrals to the hospital; and supervising distribution of medication stored in the clinic to avoid misplacement, forgetfulness, or loss. Wow! All these activities required independent judgment and highlighted the uniqueness of nursing.

Two volunteer nurses were always assigned to work together so that consulting with one another was possible. RNs with diplomas and college degrees as well as LPNs served as volunteers. Some were new graduates; others had many years of nursing experience. At the time, I was taking courses part-time toward a master's degree in community health nursing. Clinic coordinators were college graduates with liberal arts and social science degrees.

On my first day, I attended to some of the guests, most of whom were inebriated. Obtaining a history was therefore a challenge, as was the environment itself: sidestepping foot soak basins and listening to heart and lung sounds as the overhead subway roared by outside the building. Timing was everything! As the evening unfolded, my initial impression of a chaotic place changed. Although it was indeed busy, an underlying order was present, as well as much caring. Coming to the shelter after my day job was not always easy, but I continued to volunteer in the clinic for the next two and a half decades.

Relationship-building—emphasized by Barbara on my first visit—continued as a crucial component of caregiving: the guest whose infestations had been treated by a long-time nurse volunteer would request her for another health issue. I came to know one guest well whose venous stasis ulcer dressings I changed month after month and later assisted with nursing home placement. His subsequent "escape" back to Pine Street soon after reminded me that *relationship* implied an ongoing dynamic. I made regular visits to the nursing home for many years thereafter.

Another example of the importance of relationship-building with clinic guests occurred outside the shelter. A guest whom I had known from the shelter was also seen at the Boston VA hospital where I was then working. He had just been informed of his positive HIV status and responded by running down the hospital corridor sobbing and screaming, police in pursuit. Recognizing me, he calmed down. I brought him into an empty exam room after informing the police that I could handle the situation. We talked about the meaning of the lab test results, the way his illness would be addressed, and we agreed to talk later that week at the shelter clinic. He left with a semblance of hope, and I was grateful that I had been there for him. After that incident, I requested and received liaison status (between the VA Hospital and Pine Street Shelter) that enabled me to assist VA staff with other issues involving shelter guests.

One mentally ill guest presented to the clinic with an infected leg wound after falling. We were also concerned because he had stopped taking his psychoactive medication. Since he was not a serious threat to himself or others at the time, "watchful waiting" was the course. Several days passed and he experienced dramatic, worsening changes in his wound accompanied by a high fever. We feared sepsis, and he finally agreed to go to the hospital, but only if I accompanied him. However, he was unwilling to be seen at the facility where he was known; he wanted to go to the one where he was born. So off we went to his birthplace hospital. I expected trouble and we got it. Providers in the emergency room were terse, insensitive, and not pleased with our choice to be there. They seemed to ignore his poor mental state, focusing instead on his physical symptoms, which they believed were not that serious. No attempt was made to treat this man as an individual in need, much less establish a patient–provider relationship. A nursing school classmate happened to be on duty and stopped by to see me. When I told him why we were at this particular facility, he intervened and my patient was admitted.

CONTINUITY OF CARE

Continuity of care was—and is—especially important with this vulnerable population. It was addressed through documentation in guests' charts and logs reporting on symptoms such as cough, rash, or intestinal problem in order to track potential communicable disease outbreaks. Rounds were made at the hospital where most guests were admitted and concrete discharge plans were formulated after discussion with staff and guest. The clinic coordinator assisted with coordination of care, which included contacting outside agencies to make appointments, determining health insurance coverage, and scheduling volunteers.

Crossing paths with shelter guests happened regularly when I worked at the Boston Detoxification Center and provided another source of continued care. I came to know those with uncomplicated withdrawals as well as others with more difficult experiences. I often advocated for admission, an extended stay, or a specific rehab program post-detox.

Insulin-dependent diabetes is one of the most serious health issues a homeless person faces, and continuity of care is imperative. Another nurse at the shelter (a graduate school classmate) and I decided to develop a research project targeting the group of shelter guests with this condition. To begin our needs assessment, we interviewed health care providers at several facilities in the greater Boston area who treated homeless insulin-dependent diabetics to establish estimated numbers. Although in the late 1980s, five such places offered treatment, but they were underused; staff at other facilities was frequently unaware that these resources existed. From these interviews we found that substance abuse, particularly alcohol, was the major barrier to effective management of insulin-dependent diabetes and the first issue to address to avoid life-threatening complications.

We created a flow sheet for each guest's chart designed to cover areas such as recent detox experiences, blood glucose values, proteinuria, last eye evaluation, immunizations, TB tests, and primary care appointments. From these data, clinic staff formulated care guides that were distributed at the shelter for diabetics and their caregivers. Other recommendations included presentations to staff on hyperglycemic and hypoglycemic reactions, review of Medicaid coverage, wearing a Medic Alert bracelet, and insulin dosing in privacy (to avoid syringes being used as bartering items or weapons). Our research identified existing resources to treat insulin-dependent diabetes among the homeless and led to providing additional tools for controlling the condition at Pine Street and other clinics.

STUDENT LEARNING

Pine Street provided placement opportunities for college students interested in health careers. Nursing, medical, dental, and optometry students came to the shelter clinic with their faculty and interacted with guests and staff. Guests were generous in sharing their stories and were agreeable to providing material on their lives and health conditions. As students familiarized themselves with the physical problems and their unique presentations, they also learned how homelessness contributes to these problems. It was heartening to see a reluctant or hesitant student evolve into one who was eager, self-assured, and had a positive attitude toward the homeless. Some returned to volunteer, having formed relationships with the clinic and its guests.

RECIPROCITY

During my time at the shelter, I saw that reciprocity is as important to a homeless person as it is to the rest of us. Guests were aware that clinic services were free and that nurses volunteered their time. They sometimes offered tokens of appreciation, such as the day's newspaper, a candy bar, or a compliment, which we accepted. There were limits, however, when it was obvious that an item had substantial value (a piece of jewelry or clothing with price tag still attached), and we had to decline the offering. Reciprocity could also be seen in particular actions. For example, one evening after clinic hours, I found my car blocked by another vehicle in the parking lot. Some of the guests whom I knew and had cared for were standing nearby and asked why I was returning to the shelter. I pointed to my blocked car as I headed back inside to have the car's owner paged. Upon returning, I realized that the blocking vehicle had been lifted out of my way by the guests. I thanked and scolded them all in the same breath; they had risked serious injury. Above and beyond was an understatement!

A GROWING NEED

During the 1970s and 1980s, several factors combined to increase the number of homeless persons. In addition to conflicting political and financial factors facing contemporary urban centers in regard to affordable housing, deinstitutionalization of the mentally ill as well as gentrification led to a dramatic increase in homelessness. During this period, it became clear that a larger shelter was needed by Pine Street. And so, the facility bordering Chinatown moved to larger quarters in the same neighborhood (the South End) in 1980. A parade took place on moving day, complete with banners, staff, and many of the guests. We continued the same services in the new clinic, including foot soaks in the common area, having learned the benefits of this communal experience. Clinic hours expanded, a morning clinic was added, and employees were hired to accommodate increasing numbers of guests.

LOSS

Rarely does a homeless person live past age 50; life on the streets takes a hard toll. Both Barbara McInnis and one of the psychiatric nurses at the shelter realized the impact of loss on guests, and memorial services were introduced at Pine Street Inn. At these services, brightly colored crepe paper was strewn along the front fence. Cards with the name of the deceased guest were read aloud and distributed for remembrance by those attending the service. Music was provided by staff, and all were invited to share thoughts about a guest they may have known. This annual event provided an opportunity for closure and a reminder that those who had been known at Pine Street Inn were cared about and not forgotten.

ACTIVISM

Homelessness is an independent risk factor for increased morbidity and mortality. It became frustrating to see rising numbers of homeless people and less and less affordable housing in Boston. This reality led to my involvement with Housing Now, a political action group focused on housing and homelessness. I was arrested twice during demonstrations. The first occurred during a nationwide demonstration in 1986 to alert the country to the state of homelessness at the time. The judge sentenced us to 6 months' probation and after his ruling he encouraged us to "stay in trouble." My second arrest in 1987 was related to the possibility that the Massachusetts legislature would lower subsidized housing allowances. We were arrested in the State House, in the Hall of Nurses. I may not have been on the right side of the law that day but I believe the Spirit of Nurses Past supported our action.

Pine Street Shelter had always been interested in developing permanent housing for the homeless. The community in which I lived was one locale that the shelter was considering. I had had an 11-year association with the shelter at that time and knew that the homeless persons being considered for permanent housing were individuals having strong self-care abilities, not those physically or mentally unstable. The latter would strain the town's resources, with attendant fears of bringing disease and littering streets with empty liquor bottles. I testified on behalf of the shelter at a town meeting. Subsequently, the Board of Selectmen and town meeting members approved Pine Street's plan to purchase affordable housing in the community.

SELF-CARE

By the 1980s, the goal of self-care was gradually being realized by some Pine Street guests, and the opportunity to be involved in this purposeful activity was before us. Ft. Point Shelter, a facility under the umbrella of Pine Street Inn, was about to open and was seeking staff for the clinic. I very much enjoyed my independent practice at Pine Street, but here was a chance to organize a clinic from the ground up. I applied for and received the position of head nurse.

Guests staying at this shelter were expected to function at a higher level than those at Pine Street. They were younger, healthier, and some were substance-free and sober. They had jobs, bank accounts, and were saving for housing. Most believed their stay at the shelter was temporary, and they were anxious to be on their way; to be independent. Because many of their health issues, such as bronchitis, obesity, and seasonal allergies were now being monitored or were resolving, self-care was a realistic goal.

The Ft. Point Shelter was also located in the South End neighborhood of Boston, a few blocks from Pine Street. The clinic was created on the first floor of an old converted manufacturing building in a large, freshly painted space with a bathroom and two private exam rooms. Volunteers had loaned laminated posters of the old masters Monet, Van Gogh, and Degas to grace the walls. It was satisfying to offer guests a pleasant environment in which to be seen! Acute and episodic care such as first aid for falls, seizures, and referrals for detox continued to take significant clinic time, but because Pine Street tried to steer a more stable guest population to Ft. Point, we were able to focus more on health prevention issues such as updating immunizations, vision testing, and screening for head and neck cancer.

My concern for preventative health once turned into a debate with Ft. Point Shelter administration over proposed installation of cigarette and soft drink vending machines. Guests had requested that these items be made available to them, and I learned inadvertently that the topic was on the agenda of a meeting to which I had not been invited. Nonetheless, I appeared and addressed the adverse effects on health of smoking and high-sugar-content drinks, ignoring the fact that my input had not been requested. Administration agreed to cancel the cigarette machine but not the soft drink dispenser. Not everything, but it was a start toward changing attitudes of those in charge to value professional knowledge when making health care decisions.

THE FIRST LICENSED NURSE'S CLINIC IN THE UNITED STATES

Nursing interventions at both Pine Street and Ft. Point Shelters were certainly valuable but all were not billable. Five shelters with clinics were in operation by the late 1980s. Medicaid informed us that clinic licensure was a prerequisite for any reimbursement. After much hard work by many nurses inside and outside the shelters, the clinics became licensed in 1996—*the first independent nurses' clinic in the country to do so*. Licensure provided authenticity to what we had been doing for years. At the licensure celebration, former U.S. Secretary of Health and Human Services Donna Shalala described us as combat nurses on the front lines of community health care. Her description was seconded by Senator Edward Kennedy, who was also present. We were now able to generate revenue for clinic operations!

A SHIFT IN PHILOSOPHY

In 1985, physicians started to assist at the clinic. They served as consultants to staff. They examined guests unwilling to go outside for needed follow-up treatment and evaluation. They wrote prescriptions, and completed forms requiring an MD signature. It was clear at the time, however, that the physicians were at the clinic primarily as consultants and that the relationship was intended to be mutually supportive.

The move from a nursing model to a medical model at the Pine Street clinics took place over time until a major change in direction became apparent in 2003. The stance of shelter administration was that the medical model allowed for more reimbursement. It was presented as a financial decision, even though five administrators were receiving six-figure salaries and a cash reserve of over $15 million was in place at the time, as disclosed by the *Boston Globe*. Given the circumstances, it was difficult to understand how the nurses' clinics were not affordable. Licensure was in place for Medicaid reimbursement of some services, and grants had been written to defray the cost of others. Yet these efforts were dismissed. Although building trust is not compensated for by Medicaid or other insurance plans, it is an absolute necessity for the homeless. The nursing model, based on relationship-building and trust, had worked well for 31 years. When the five nurses' clinics closed in 2003, 150,000 clinical encounters (1,250 per month) were documented, in contrast to 426 encounters recorded during Pine Street's first month of operation years ago. Shelter management did not seem to value the significance of this history nor the power of nursing in having accomplished it.

REFLECTIONS

Revisiting my 27 years with the Pine Street's nurses' clinics brings forth rich memories of people and incidents. Paul Sullivan, the first director of the Pine Street Shelter, set in motion the nurses' clinic, and his support of its concept and effectiveness was unfailing. He died in 1983 and was therefore no longer the director when administration chose to change care provision at the clinic from a nursing to a medical model. His presence was sorely missed when clinic nursing care ended. Clinic staff believed he would have been able to work out a solution to enable the clinic to continue with the nursing model in place.

Barbara McInnis, the TB Control nurse assigned to Pine Street by the Massachusetts Department of Public Health, was a role model, mentor, and the heart and soul of the nurses' clinic. She died during the transition from the nursing care model to the medical model. Although we miss her support, her influence has lived on in our professional and personal lives. Each year we celebrate her birthday, retelling "Barbara stories" and sharing what we are doing in our lives because of her.

I would be remiss if I failed to recall the dozens of dedicated clinic volunteers and staff during my long association with Pine Street Shelters. Several returned to school while working there, and after the nurses' clinic was no longer in operation they obtained additional nursing degrees as BSNs, MSNs, NPs, and PhDs; two received divinity degrees. Others became nurse educators and supervisors in local hospitals; still others pursued research endeavors. Quite a few continued to work with the homeless in other shelters and through churches. One former staff nurse opened a shelter in another state. Loyalty of clinic staff is reflected in the large numbers who began working in the early years of Pine Street's nurses' clinic and were present when it ended. This group includes two psychiatric nurses who worked there for over 25 years.

The more informal aspects of Pine Street life are also important. Lasting friendships and sometimes romances evolved among shelter staff. So many caring and creative people worked there—those in human services, artists, musicians, writers; no wonder they were drawn to one another! The clinic bulletin board displayed many happy life changes, wedding announcements, new-baby pictures, and letters from faraway places where former colleagues were expanding their Pine Street experience, taking their energies to other environments. Bonding was a powerful force.

Today there are over 250 nurse-managed clinics in the United States caring for the underserved; financed through states, charitable organizations, and federal grants. Although President Obama's 2010 Affordable Care Act authorized over $50 million for 5 years for nurse-managed clinics, only $15 million has been made available.

The need for such facilities is growing, especially because of the acute shortage of primary care physicians and the growth of underserved populations. In the 1970s, the estimated number of homeless persons in Boston was 4,000 to 6,000 (no formal census was taken in that era). In 2013, the figure was 7,255. These latest numbers do a better job of reflecting the range of services being provided to homeless individuals—in contrast with how data were collected years ago.

Accomplishments of the Pine Street nurses' clinic are many: providing skilled nursing care to vulnerable people, educating students and providers to the health needs of the homeless, and obtaining licensure, to name a few. I will always be proud of my association with Pine Street Shelter. It raised my consciousness regarding the importance of patient care, relationship-building, allowing client choice, and political action. My sadness with how the Pine Street nurse's clinic ended was assuaged by a 9-year involvement in nursing education whereby I was able to transmit the message to students that nursing care with the homeless is a joy and a privilege. Most of all, I am gratified to have participated in an effort to provide an empowering environment in which members of this vulnerable population worked to achieve self-care.

16

Serving People Living With HIV/AIDS

A World of Difference

MIKE OLUFEMI

Editor's Note: I had the pleasure of getting to know Mike Olufemi when he enrolled in the global health nursing course that I teach. Mike is originally from Nigeria. I assumed he would return to Nigeria, or another area of Africa, to meet requirements for the course. Instead, he travelled to Australia to volunteer in a clinic serving gay men living with HIV. Upon returning to school, Mike negotiated with his public health nursing instructor for a clinical placement with a local program serving people living with HIV. As an African man, Mike brings an important voice to the global discussion regarding HIV/AIDS. He begins his story by reflecting on access to health care, as he experienced it, in his childhood village.

REFLECTIONS ON HEALTH CARE IN NIGERIA

I was born in a small village in Osun State, Nigeria. Many such villages across the country lack electricity, clinics, potable water, and good roads. As a child, I remember a doctor (now I wonder if he ever went to a medical school or if he was part of a volunteer group) came once or twice a year. He simply assessed those who were ill and administered medications. The rest of the year, when villagers became critically ill, they traveled several miles, often on foot, to reach a local pharmacy in a bigger village. Although he was unlicensed, the pharmacist diagnosed their ailments and sold medications to treat their symptoms. At times, villagers sought the services of herbalists. Others, who could not afford the cost, simply relied on their own knowledge of locally available herbs. I have vivid memories of family members boiling the bark or leaves of trees, known to have medicinal properties, to treat malaria. I remember an uncle who died of pneumonia and other villagers who died from simple illnesses due to poor access to health care.

My father was the village chief and the most educated person in the community. He had a high school diploma but he did not have the financial means to further his education. When I was a boy, our small village had a primary school, constructed of mud and unevenly plastered with cheap concrete. The rooms leaked when it rained, making it difficult to teach or learn. But we were lucky to have a school when many bigger villages did not have one at all. Poverty notwithstanding, most Nigerian parents strive to educate their children because they believe that education is the gateway to prosperity.

I lost my mother when I was 10 years old; she died in a vehicle accident during one of her journeys to the city to buy merchandise for sale in the village. I was a good student in school and that could be the reason my father's stepsister invited me to live with her in the city of Ibadan after my mother's demise. Although I was in a city, health practices were similar to what I had experienced in my village except that there were pharmacies, private clinics, and hospitals.

In those years, health care was subsidized in public hospitals, although patients had to wait a long time. Today, health care is simply "cash and carry," meaning you receive services if you have the money to pay. Patients are often denied treatment if they don't have the required deposit, resulting in preventable deaths. Delays in getting to the hospital, lack of supplies, or power outages contribute to high mortality rates. Such is the deplorable state of the health care system in Nigeria today. There is also a brain drain in the country, as many doctors and other professionals leave in search of a better life abroad.

I studied chemistry at the prestigious University of Lagos in Nigeria, where I earned advanced degrees in chemical engineering and business administration. I was a chemistry teacher for about a year before joining Dunlop Nigeria Plc (a tire manufacturing and marketing company) in 1995. I was the Product Evaluation Manager for the company until March 2002 when I decided to relocate to the

United States in search of new experiences and opportunities. Like many young Africans, I became part of the brain drain.

MY PATH TO NURSING

I have an unquenchable thirst for knowledge and I love to explore new opportunities. However, I will say that circumstance drove me into the field of nursing. When I arrived in 2002 it was extremely difficult to land a manufacturing job. Relocating to the United States was like starting all over again, despite my education, work experience, and skills. The story is the same for many immigrants who take up odd jobs that are not commensurate with their qualifications and skills.

Reality forces an immigrant to choose a career that can easily guarantee a job. Nursing is one such profession. My first taste of nursing came when working part-time at Heritage Christian Services in Rochester, New York, as a resident councilor, to augment my unstable real estate commission. Initially, it was a challenge to transition from chemical engineering to caring for people who were developmentally challenged and had special needs. However, within a short period of time I became comfortable assisting patients with personal and physical care, consistent with their nursing care plans. I helped them connect with their community; taking them to church on Sundays, engaging them in recreational activities, and taking them to visit their families on weekends. It was the beginning of a new career path for me.

I enrolled in a licensed practical nursing program and worked briefly in a small community hospital before moving to North Carolina. Since 2006, I have worked in a retirement community providing direct care to residents in rehabilitation and long-term care settings. Because I love what I do I decided to become a professional nurse. I get personal satisfaction from helping others reach their health and wellness potential and felt that a professional degree in nursing would provide a greater ability to do so.

GLOBAL HEALTH AND HIV/AIDS

When I entered the nursing program, I was delighted to learn about global health opportunities. I seized on the opportunity to travel. I realized that global health studies would give me a new perspective on health care systems in other areas of the world. Growing up in Nigeria exposed me to the plight of people living in abject poverty, lack of basic infrastructure, lack of access to health care, and the social isolation of people living with diseases such as HIV/AIDS. I was interested in how these social determinants of health would compare in a developed nation. I chose to go to Australia because I was interested in learning how its health care system differs in comparison to the United States, since Australia has successfully implemented Universal Health Care.

VICTORIA AIDS COUNCIL/GAY MEN'S HEALTH CENTRE

I elected to complete my global health experience with the Victorian AIDS Council/Gay Men's Health Centre (VAC/GMHC) in Melbourne. I learned about the organization through online searches during the initial stage of the planning process. The Centre Clinic—one program of the VAC/GMHC—is located above a pharmacy with the entrance at the back of the building to provide privacy to its clients. I worked with two practice nurses (the equivalent of RNs in the United States) and doctors (often referred to as general practitioners [GPs]) who consulted with patients who primarily were HIV positive and homosexual. The clinic provides sexually transmitted infection (STI) screening, treatment, and support to people living with HIV (PLHIV). Vaccinations were also administered to those at risk for hepatitis, pneumonia, and so on.

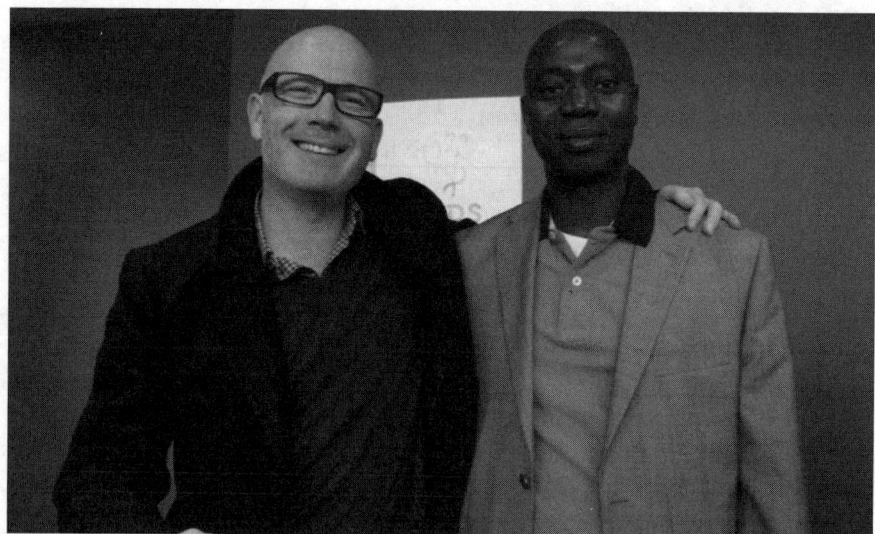

Figure 16.1 Simon Powell, manager, clinical services, VAC/GMHC and Mike Olufemi.

There were a number of ongoing research studies in which some of the patients were enrolled, and specific labs and follow-up data were often collected during their appointment at the clinic. Education is also a key aspect of the nursing function. The majority of the clients were middle class and well educated. Therefore, sharing information about lab results, such as viral loads and CD4 counts with HIV positive patients, was relatively easy. Education about adherence to medication regimen to prevent drug resistance, sexual practices, and the need for protection to prevent transmission is routinely provided at the clinic. Also informing newly diagnosed HIV clients about resources available to them in the community is important. It was amazing to see many PLHIV/AIDS that were in good health with the help of antiretroviral therapy and the combined efforts of doctors, nurses, support services, and positive living by the patients.

I spent 2 days with the Positive Living Center (PLC), another program of the VAC/GMHC, which occupies an old library in South Yarra. The PLC provides integrated and comprehensive services, including a program designed to address nutritional, legal, housing, recreational, and other needs of PLHIV/AIDS in the state of Victoria. I had a wonderful experience working with two nurses from the Royal District Nursing Service (RDNS). The RDNS provides 24/7 home care to patients on a one-on-one basis to promote independence and advocacy for their clients. RDNS specializes in medication, wound and diabetes management, aged and palliative care, HIV/AIDS, and hospital in the home (HITH). I also spent time in other agencies with which the VAC/GMHC has collaborative arrangements.

NURSING SKILLS

At the Centre Clinic, I was able to utilize my nursing skills by assisting the GPs and the RNs in taking vital signs, drawing labs for several tests such as viral loads, CD4 levels, kidney and liver function tests, as well as throat and anal swabs for STI screening, gonorrhea, and chlamydia in particular. I also helped in taking patients' weights and administering injections such as vitamin B_{12}. I worked with an RDNS district nurse visiting patients in their homes. Most of these clients had complex medical conditions, such as mental health needs, domestic violence, diabetes, and drugs and/or alcohol issues, in addition to having HIV/AIDS. The district nurse assists clients with housing needs, medication administration, diabetes management, nutrition, health promotion initiatives, as well as many nonmedical issues.

The other RDNS nurse works out of the Victoria Infectious Disease Service (VIDS) clinic at the Royal Melbourne Hospital. This arrangement is an indication of the level of collaboration among health care organizations in Victoria. The nurse spent a lot of time educating clients about health promotion initiatives. Many of the patients engaged me in conversations about their health, and the wonderful roles nurses play in managing their anxiety and apprehension when diagnosed with HIV. Others initiated conversations about the United States, and Africa, with topics ranging from health care to politics.

DIFFICULT DECISIONS AND CHOICES

I interacted with a number of clients facing difficult decisions and choices, including a young gay man who had immigrated to Australia to join his partner. HIV testing is mandatory for people filing for permanent residency in Australia. Unfortunately, he tested positive for HIV. He had the opportunity to get free medical care elsewhere, but preferred to come to the Centre Clinic, where he was required to pay for his visits, labs, treatments, and medications. His decision was based on perceived confidentiality and privacy concerns. On top of that was the fear of stigma, discrimination, and social isolation he might face in his community. He avoided going to the Centre Clinic regularly for routine labs because of cost.

At one point, I was introduced to a refugee woman who was HIV positive. I was told that the patient would only see the same nurse and/or doctor during her visits to the clinic, and that she had refused treatment for about a year. She was also reported to have been alienated from her small immigrant community when it was suspected she had been going to the infectious disease clinic. Even though she was provided with alternative accommodation elsewhere, she was reported to be in distress because she missed living among her people.

In another case, a patient was faced with the dilemma of not wanting his wife to know he had tested positive for HIV but at the same time wanting to make sure she was tested and not infected. After much soul searching, and discussions with clinic staff, the patient arrived at a solution. Ultimately, his wife was tested and found to be negative. The patient returned to the clinic overjoyed by the news and stated that he felt as if a big load had been lifted from his shoulders. However, the underlying ethical issue regarding full disclosure of the patient's HIV status to his wife was not resolved.

As these stories demonstrate, nurses play a vital role in ensuring the overall well-being of their patients. It is particularly crucial to connect with PLHIV/AIDS through therapeutic communication: acknowledging their problems, showing empathy, and remaining nonjudgmental. As the case of the HIV-positive husband illustrates, nurses also have the responsibility of advocating for not just their patients but also others that may be impacted by their patients' actions or inactions.

DIFFERENT STROKES AND GLOBAL STRIDES

My professional goal for this experience had been to broaden my understanding of HIV/AIDS health policies in regard to prevention, health promotion, education, and community response to HIV in Australia as compared to the United States and parts of Africa. As anticipated, Australia provided me with a new perspective; one that was different from what I had been exposed to in Africa and in the United States.

Australia

Australia, with a population of approximately 22.5 million, has about 22,000 PLHIV/AIDS. The prevalence is low among heterosexuals and also among drug-injecting individuals. Therefore, in Australia, attention is focused more on gay men because they are intrinsically linked to increased HIV incidence. The state of Victoria in particular focuses on prevention among the most stigmatized groups, including gay men, culturally diverse groups, and women (Victoria AIDS Council 2011–12 Annual Report). I think that the Universal Health Care system in Australia is of great help to PLHIV. Treatment is affordable and prevention takes utmost priority.

The United States

The United States presents a slightly different HIV/AIDS picture when compared to Australia. According to the Centers for Disease Control and Prevention (CDC), the United States, with a population of 314 million, has an estimated 1.15 million people living with HIV infection (CDC.org). An estimated 50,000 new cases of HIV occur in the United States annually, a number that has remained stable over recent years. Most affected are gay, bisexual, and other men who have sex with men (MSM) of all races. Meanwhile, African Americans and Hispanics are disproportionally affected and severely impacted by the infection. In 2010, Blacks, who make up 12% of the U.S. population, accounted for 44% of new HIV infections. Hispanics, with 16% of the U.S. population, accounted for 21% of new cases in the same year (CDC.org). Recent trends also reveal that young African American MSM aged 12 to 24 have the highest rate of new HIV infection. This is a disturbing trend indeed.

Socioeconomic disparities (access to health care, employment opportunities, education, and housing) are key determinants of health faced by minority groups. Unlike Australia with its Universal Health Care system, the United States struggles with how best to address high rates of uninsured people and mounting health care costs.

After returning from Australia, I had an opportunity to volunteer with the Alliance of AIDS Services Carolina (AASC), a nonprofit organization dedicated to HIV prevention, education, and advocacy for PLHIV/AIDS. The AASC is one of several local organizations that provide housing, spiritual support, financial support, and affordable treatment options for PLHIV/AIDS. This range of services is similar to what I observed in Melbourne.

While enrolled in my undergraduate public health nursing course, I conducted a survey with two other classmates to explore and evaluate resources available to PLHIV/AIDS in Durham County, North Carolina. We found that many of the agencies that serve this population were saddled with limited resources and poor coordination, resulting in their efforts not being appropriately channeled to reach the most at-risk populations.

Africa

While in Melbourne, it was difficult not to compare attitudes and beliefs with those held in my home country.

Homosexuality is a very volatile issue in Nigeria, especially in the northern part of the country where Islamic laws are strictly enforced. Jail terms await those found guilty in sharia courts. The southern and western regions of the country are more liberal due to Western influence. However, a majority of Christians living in those areas also frown on homosexuality. I stayed in the home of Nigerian friends during my visit to Melbourne. My choice to volunteer with the Gay Men's Health Centre caused a contentious argument with my friend's wife about homosexuality. She was not as open-minded and accepting of homosexuality as I thought she would be considering her university education. My friend, on the other hand, avoided the topic entirely. Millions of Nigerians fall into these two categories: those who vehemently oppose homosexuality and those who do not want to be dragged into such a contentious debate.

HIV/AIDS is another sensitive issue in Nigeria. Some people in Africa still believe that HIV is a myth and others think it is a design by the Western world to get rid of Black people. People are scared to be tested because of the social stigma associated with the infection. Furthermore, treatment eludes most as a result of the exorbitant cost of antiretroviral therapy (ART).

In 2011, an estimated 34 million people were living with HIV globally while sub-Saharan Africa accounted for 69% of that number (who.org). In my birth country of Nigeria it is estimated that about 3.6% of the population is living with HIV/AIDS (avert.org). Several thousand people die of AIDS annually, many of whom were not even diagnosed (life expectancy is only 52 years in Nigeria compared to 78 years in the United States).

One thing is certain; poverty is a major health determinant in most parts of Africa. Education is grossly lacking in regard to sexual transmission, vertical transmission, and AIDS-related maternal mortality, intolerance for gender-based violence, and tuberculosis (TB) deaths (unaids.org). The good news is that new HIV infection is declining globally, as is the number of children infected with HIV and people dying of AIDS-related causes. Increased access to ART has helped to alleviate the burden of infection in sub-Saharan Africa. However, it is worthy to note that stigma and discrimination continue to impede effective HIV response in many countries, even in developed countries like Australia and the U.S. prevention strategies have been hampered by sex practices, risk behaviors, and the dynamic nature of social interactions among gay men in Australia and the United States in particular.

IMPLICATIONS FOR NURSING PRACTICE

My trip to Australia was a worthwhile experience. I learned the importance of serving people living with HIV/AIDS while acknowledging their problems, showing empathy, and remaining nonjudgmental. I participated in the care of HIV patients using approaches tailored to meet their specific needs. I witnessed collaborative teamwork within and among various support and advocacy groups, health care organizations, the academic community, clinical research organizations, and volunteers; all of whom focused on preventing the transmission of HIV/STIs and caring for PLHIV/AIDS. Overall, the experience helped me integrate global health concepts with the health care practices I observed and participated in while in Melbourne. The trip helped me understand and compare cultural and health practices in Australia with those of the United States and parts of Africa. It offered me the opportunity to gain exposure to professional nursing, coordinated health care, and support services for PLHIV/AIDS.

My volunteer work with the Alliance of AIDS Services Carolina gave me an opportunity to interact with HIV agencies and HIV-positive clients in my local community. These experiences exposed me to the dynamics in play at the local and state level regarding prevention, treatment, and advocacy for PLHIV/AIDS.

My background as a Nigerian, informed by my volunteer experiences in Australia and Durham, has instilled in me a desire to address the devastation of HIV/AIDS in Africa. I feel compelled to give back to a continent that is ravaged by war, disease, and abject poverty. There are complex sociocultural and political dynamics in Africa that slow efforts to curtail the spread of HIV. I believe that Africans, in the diaspora, have a unique vantage point from which to navigate these waters. I hope to join an international organization involved in HIV prevention and treatment so that I can return to sub-Saharan Africa to serve those with the greatest need.

REFERENCES

AVERT (2013). HIV and AIDS in Nigeria: 2012 Statistics. Retrieved from http://www.avert.org

CDC (2013). HIV in the United States: At A Glance. Retrieved from http://www.cdc.org

UNAIDS (2013). UNAIDS Strategy 2011–2015. Retrieved from http://www.unaids.org

Victoria AIDS Council 2011–12 Annual Report.

WHO (2013). HIV/AIDS: Global Situation and Trends. Retrieved from http://www.who.org

III

Global Health Nursing in Research and Consultation

Sharing Knowledge

The final section in this collection of narratives continues with nurses who describe themselves as teachers, researchers, and consultants. In doing so, they illustrate important contributions to our body of knowledge regarding best practices in global health nursing.

17

With Real Heart

Nursing and Midwifery in Latin America

JENNIFER FOSTER

Editor's Note: Jennifer Foster shares her path to global health with wonderful detail about her Peace Corps experience and her decision to continue her career as a nurse midwife and later into academia. Jenny continues her narrative by describing her community-based participatory research conducted in the Dominican Republic and discusses the relationships and strategies she used to assure sustainability for the program. She reflects on her journey in which she moved from being a nurse who cares for individual women across the globe to one who cares for the nurses and midwives who care for individual women across the globe.

GETTING THERE

Though I was completely unaware at the time, my path to becoming a global nurse began when I was swimming in the ocean, where I grew up on Long Island, New York. It was a hot, summer day between senior year in high school and freshman year in college. I was with a friend I hadn't seen in a long time, and we were comparing our dreams while jumping over the breaking waves, imagining what we would like to see, and to do, in life. I had completed my third year of high school Spanish and I told my friend I wanted to go to South America. The whole South American continent seemed so exotic and compelling. Surprisingly, my friend said her family knew a pediatric researcher at Johns Hopkins University who was half Peruvian and studied malnutrition in children in Lima. She offered to speak with him about my volunteering with his project, and perhaps being able to live with a family. I was drawn to the idea of serving the poor in a foreign place.

So, in the summer of 1971, I spent 8 weeks in Lima, Peru. I lived with a Peruvian family, and I volunteered at the Anglo American Hospital in Lima, where the physician friend was conducting longitudinal research. His study followed children who had been hospitalized for kwashiorkor and marasmus, rehabilitated, and sent home to their families who had been taught to add protein-fortified flour to their children's food. The study tracked the children's anthropometric profiles for 5 years after they had been rehabilitated. Over the summer, I accompanied a wonderful Peruvian woman who was his research assistant in the project. She collected data on the children at home, year after year.

My eyes were opened to the breadth of poverty and inequality in health in South America. I had never seen people picking through garbage to find food. It never occurred to me then to pursue a health career, but I was forever transformed by bearing witness to such poverty. After the summer, I began my college career at Harvard. I pursued botany, and Latin American history and literature. I was successful academically but—after a summer spent with children who were stunted from malnutrition—I found the affluence of Harvard and the self-satisfaction of many Harvard students alienating. I knew I wanted to study something with human applicability. It never occurred to me then to study medicine or nursing. Premed students at Harvard, at that time, were busy destroying lab notes of their classmates to make sure they beat them at getting in to medical school—not my style. I had successfully internalized the ideology of patriarchy—nursing seemed an alien and (or so I thought then) inferior profession, because it was dominated by women, and I thought everyone worked in hospitals—also not my style.

I learned I did not want to become a literary scholar, and I wasn't happy at Harvard. I decided to take a year off after my sophomore year. I was privileged to have my parents agree, albeit reluctantly. My father was a Harvard graduate, as were many relatives since the 1600s, including my brother and later, my sister. My ancestors were Boston Brahmin, and my great-grandmother's sister was married to J.P. Morgan. My father was afraid I would never return to Harvard, and his fear was realized, because I never did.

In the summer after my sophomore year in college, I volunteered for the American Friends Service Committee in Mexico, working with a team of Mexican and U.S. students to build latrines in a rural village. We built latrines, and we also did what the Mexican villagers really wanted: we helped build a wall around their cemetery so that the donkeys wouldn't poop on their graves. Every Wednesday morning, a Mexican physician traveled to the village to hold a clinic. The village had no electricity or running water. Tuesday nights, people would begin to line up to see the doctor the next morning. Inevitably, as the Wednesday morning session ended, not all the people had been seen. Some of them needed follow up. The doctor asked for volunteers to change bandages, check on vomiting children, and see that medicine had been taken. I volunteered.

One day, I walked home through a cornfield to get back to the school (our dormitory). I had just checked the wound of a woman who had accidently lacerated her foot with the axe she was using to chop wood to heat her stove. I had an epiphany. I knew my life's calling was to become a nurse, a public health nurse. I wanted to visit people in their homes and help them recover. The profession that had previously been so alien and inferior suddenly opened up to me: I would do whatever was required to enter it.

I transferred from Harvard to the BSN program at the University of Rochester (NY), where I graduated in 1976. For the most part, I really liked nursing school, even though no nursing student is willing to admit they like nursing school. I believe I got a good education in nursing. I knew I wanted to go into public health, but in those years, nurses insisted one must begin a career with hospital work experience, so I worked on an oncology unit for a year. Twelve months to the day after I began working in the hospital, I resigned and joined the Peace Corps, assigned to Guatemala for 2 years.

GLOBAL NURSING

Clinical Practice

My global practice of nursing includes both clinical and research experiences. These experiences have been constitutive of my identity as a global nurse. How do I define a global nurse? In my view, a global nurse is a nurse whose vision and perspective is oriented to the health and well-being of all peoples, wherever they live on earth. Given that the poorest people bear a disproportionate burden of illness and premature death, global nurses often focus upon communities, populations, or regions that are poor economically. Poverty can be found in all nations, and varies in population pockets within nations. However, in general, the distribution of poverty around the world is concentrated in the global south. My Peace Corps assignment was an experiential lesson in the poverty of the global south.

My most significant clinical work as a global nurse was in the rural, western highlands of indigenous Guatemala. I worked as the only graduate-trained nurse in a health post that served surrounding villages of 5,000 Kaqchikel Mayans. The Guatemalan staff consisted of two auxiliary nurses, a social worker, and a physician that came from Guatemala City a few days a week. Most of the male villagers spoke Spanish and Kaqchikel. Most of the women spoke Kaqchikel only. The village was about 15 miles from the paved Pan American Highway (a two-lane road at that time), and we had electricity from 6 p.m. to 9 p.m. every evening. The evening ritual was the Mayor's walk to the generator, to start the electricity for the evening.

I lived alone, in a house made of pressed plywood: the earthquake of 1976 had destroyed the adobe houses in the village, and pressed wood and tin provided by the Canadian government provided supposedly temporary housing. Like many towns after disasters, though, temporary housing became permanent housing. I worked in the clinic from 8 a.m. till noon, and 2 p.m. till 6 p.m., Monday to Friday. When the physician was not present (most of the time), my work was much like a nurse practitioner. Unfortunately, I did not yet have the training to practice as a nurse practitioner.

Nevertheless, I was the most trained person there when the physician was absent, and I set about to learn as much as I could to give the best care I could. We reused disposable needles and sterilized them in a pressure cooker. I sutured wounds when I had no other person to do it. I leaned on the Hesperian Foundation's, *Donde No Hay Doctor* (Lerner, 1977). Mostly I insisted on being kind to people who came to the clinic, even when we had little to offer them. We were always running out of drugs. The Ministry of Health sent medications every 3 months, but never enough to last until the next shipment. So many decisions had to be made between the lesser of two bad choices: do we give a full course of antibiotics to a few, or a lesser course to more people? How do we refuse an IV to those who were convinced it was the only thing that would restore their strength, when they had walked 16 kilometers to be seen? I refused to turn people away, although the auxiliary nurses were upset with villagers who did not keep the clinic schedule. I lived in the village, so I was reachable at night when there was an emergency.

One of the components of my job description was to "supervise" the traditional midwives, or *comadronas.* Births took place at home with a local comadrona. They were women from the village who were trusted, without formal education or training. My baccalaureate degree in nursing had prepared me minimally to assist in hospital deliveries; I had nothing of the experience of the comadronas. "Supervising" included monthly continuing education meetings, to discuss births and family planning methods they could recommend to the women under their care. Mostly, the comadronas were amused by me. I was unmarried and childless, and therefore, in their view, not credible on matters of birth. Nevertheless, I held them with great respect and tried my best to speak Kaqchikel with them. We shared a mutually high regard for each other and laughed at lot together.

At the time of my arrival in the village, the 15 comadronas of the surrounding villages had recently received Ministry of Health training funded by UNICEF. The training focused on clean delivery and when to refer to the health center. At the end of the training, they received a black bag with equipment for a clean delivery: clamp, scissors, soap, apron, placenta basin, towels. This bag was a source of great pride to the comadronas. Some of them did not use it because they did not want it to get dirty. One comadrona wanted it to be buried with her upon her death.

In time, the comadronas came to trust me more and more, and sometimes called upon me at night if they needed help with a delivery. I remember vividly my sweaty hands and the pit in my stomach when I heard a knock on my door one night, with a father asking me to come help the midwife. I lit a candle, dressed quickly, and flipped through the relevant pages of *Donde No Hay Doctor*, praying everything would be alright. When I got to the house, the baby delivered shortly thereafter, without complications. The family and the comadrona were convinced I had done something marvelous. I had done nothing. But I knew then I wanted to get the training to really know what to do. I wanted to become a midwife. As a trained midwife, one could have a positive impact on women and their families, by being there, but with knowledge. Years later, after I had become a midwife, I came to realize that the baby who delivered quickly after I had arrived at the family's house had probably been occiput posterior and finally rotated to occiput anterior, making delivery straightforward. The power of helping the mother feel supported helped that to happen, too.

Thirty-five years ago, Guatemala did not have the workforce to employ graduate nurses in the rural health posts, which is how I came to work there as a Peace Corps nurse. Now, there are Guatemalan nurses staffing these facilities, and it would be much more unusual for a U.S. graduate nurse to practice clinically in a government-run health center. Many of these Guatemalan nurses speak the indigenous language of their community. Obviously this will vary from country to country, but in general, graduate nurses are more plentiful in many developing countries today. I look back on those years as ones in which I was able to provide the best service I could within the constraints of the environment. The experience definitely confirmed my passion for a global focus thereafter.

When I returned to the United States, I pursued a master's in public health degree and certification as a nurse-midwife. My purpose was to improve the care of poor women. Over the course of the next 20 years, I practiced midwifery in rural Mississippi, Maryland, Molokai (Hawaii), and in a Puerto Rican community in western Massachusetts. Even though I did not work globally, my sensibilities were global, from urban Holyoke, Massachusetts to rural Kaunakakai, Hawaii. When our two sons were grown, I was able to refocus outside the United States.

When our youngest son was six, I had returned to school to pursue a doctorate in cultural anthropology. Many of the most pressing and intractable public health problems in maternal-newborn health, it seemed to me, were related to culture. Not just the culture of patients, but also, especially, the culture of doctors, nurses, and health systems. Anthropology asks interesting, provocative questions that can become applied to health research. This type of research has a name in the health sciences literature: implementation science.

> Implementation science is the study of methods to promote the integration of research findings and evidence into healthcare policy and practice. It seeks to understand the behavior of healthcare professionals and other stakeholders as a key variable in the sustainable uptake, adoption, and implementation of evidence-based interventions. (Fogarty International Center, 2013)

I realized by the time I finished my PhD in 2003 that I had transitioned from a nurse who cared for individual women across the globe to one who cares for *the nurses and midwives* who care for individual women across the globe. That transition has taken a turn toward public health, nursing leadership, and research. The following section describes my experience in global nursing/anthropology research.

Research Practice

Shortly after I completed my PhD, a midwife colleague, Annie Heath, returned from several years teaching in the midwifery program at the University of Puerto Rico. Annie came to me with an idea for global collaboration. While in Puerto Rico, she had been invited to provide consultation in the Dominican Republic with a group of nurses from a referral hospital in the northeast of the country. The Dominican nurses were distressed because of an increase in maternal deaths on their maternity unit. Six women had died on their unit in the last 6 months of 2002, whereas three had died in the whole year of 2001. The nurses asked for a *diagnóstico* [assessment] of the situation, as well as consultation to prevent future maternal deaths. At the nurses' request, Annie planned a series of educational conferences in their hospital. Over the next 3 years, midwives from the United States, along with other nurses and physicians, taught week-long educational conferences providing the core content of midwifery to the nurses who attended the vaginal deliveries in the hospital. The nurses attended classes in the morning and practiced their new clinical skills in the afternoon. Annie asked me if I would develop a research component to the project. To understand how my research evolved in the Dominican Republic, it is important to understand the background that enabled the development of a research infrastructure at that site. It began first as a program of clinical educational conferences and evolved into a Dominican U.S. nursing project, the ADAMES project, which is briefly described here.

In 2004, Annie created a private, nonprofit organization, "Proyecto ADAMES," whose mission is to reduce maternal mortality in the Dominican hospital where the nurses first asked for consultation. By design, in 2011, the U.S. incorporation of Proyecto ADAMES closed, and the project's assets were transferred to the Associación ADAMES, which is financially partnered with the Dominican nonprofit, la Asociación Internacional de Caridad, Dominican chapter. Decisions about the project's direction, activities, and finances are now made by a Dominican executive board of nurses and other community leaders active with the hospital. By transferring actual ownership to the Dominicans, the intent is to build leadership capacity within the nurses to manage the project.

My research involvement with Proyecto ADAMES began in 2004 with a formative study to evaluate the knowledge, skills, and attitudes of the nurses who had attended the educational conferences conducted by the project (Foster, Regueira, Burgos, & Sanchez, 2005). The study used the anthropology rapid assessment process, which is an iterative qualitative process, interviewing both insiders and outsiders to evaluate a situation. I needed a Dominican partner to assist me in the project, and I turned to the nurses involved in Proyecto ADAMES to help me locate one. One of the nurses who used to be the sub Director of Nursing for the hospital, but who had become a professor of nursing at the local campus of the large, land grant university, Universidad Autónoma de Santo Domingo, had some names to suggest.

I interviewed the first person she suggested, a very formal, business-like woman, asking a high fee for her work. I knew intuitively this person was not the right person to be my research partner. As an anthropologist, I wanted to delve deeply into the situation and not take a detached approach. I asked the nursing professor, Rosa Burgos, if she would be willing to be my research partner. She agreed, and this partnership has lasted 9 years at the time of this writing. It has been a rich, educational, and very complex experience. In the following section, I detail the complexities of doing cross-cultural research, and how I have (imperfectly) navigated that path.

After the evaluation project was completed, the next study focused upon assessing the decision-making process of the nurses in the maternity ward, who had already received training through the ADAMES project. This study used another anthropological method, Decision Tree Modeling, (Gladwin, 1989), in which the researcher identifies how a cultural group (in this case a group of nurses on the maternity ward) made decisions about management of postpartum bleeding. The findings of this study revealed that knowledge of the appropriate management of postpartum hemorrhage was not a problem among the nurses.

Rather, the problem was that a sense of accountability to routinely, proactively assess for bleeding was not part of the organizational culture (Foster, Regueira, & Heath, 2006). Thus nurses were not oriented to providing the care they knew how to give, because the hospital was not oriented toward "patient-centered care." Patient-centered care is a term currently used in the quality and safety education for health professionals' movement in the United States (Cronenwett et al., 2007).

The findings of the decision tree study provided an "aha" moment for me: knowledge about providing good obstetrical care has been delivered over and over in global conferences, workshops, trainings, and consultations. But the real issue is: *How can nurses and other health providers work together globally to sustain motivation to give good care (care they know how to provide), in the context of great resource constraints?* This question has become the driving query behind the research I have conducted and plan to conduct in the future.

Resource constraints in the developing world context are a huge drain on personnel morale. Resource constraints can be material, such as insufficient supplies or space. Constraints can also be due to inadequate staffing, as the history of global health care workforce shortages attests (Joint Learning Initiative, 2004). One of the most important constraints, however, relates to the sustained drive to provide good nursing, midwifery, and medical practice. This is a place where global nurses have much to contribute, as well as much to learn, to make an impact.

In many places around the globe, good nursing and midwifery practice is unappreciated, while nurses and midwives with poor practice are not held accountable. Since history, politics, and organizational cultures vary globally, it is impossible, as well as morally questionable, for nurses from the outside, coming from a place of privilege (usually the global north), to judge or to criticize practice. Often, a nurse who considers himself/herself a global nurse educator or researcher may have a grant or special project in another country, and when that grant or project ends, so does the participation in that country. It is easy for the local nurses, and the people who they take care of, to believe that making changes, or implementing new practices, depends on people from the outside, not from within themselves. Thus, the status quo is perpetuated (Kretzmann & McKnight, 1993). Real change happens from within, from the people who want change to happen. Education is the liberating force for change, as Paulo Freire discovered, as community people become conscious of their own oppression and realize they can become agents of change for themselves (Freire, 1971).

On the other hand, nurses working globally can serve to inspire and motivate nurses in low-resource settings to discover how they can rightfully improve the conditions of their workplace and their patients. Global nurses do this by sharing knowledge resources, true collaboration, and moral support. They can encourage leadership among local nurses for positive practice change in their own context. To be successful, this requires a great deal of cultural humility and a long-term commitment to a specific site (Foster, 2009). It also demands an authentic commitment to power sharing.

The best research approach to sharing power is community-based participatory research (CBPR), which has been defined as a "collaborative research approach designed to ensure and establish structures for participation by communities affected by the issue being studied, representatives of organizations, and researchers in all aspects of the research process to improve health and well-being through taking action, including social change" (Viswanathan et al., 2004, p. 3).

The idea to conduct a CBPR study with the Dominican nurses came out of a desire for a collaborative research project that would encourage the nurses to be involved in every aspect of the research, as well as to listen to the community in ways that were impossible in the current organizational structure. One of the questions that the nurses repeatedly asked was, "Why do women wait until they are so sick to come to the hospital?" This became the research question for the CBPR study we conducted from 2008 to 2011.

To answer the question, we formed a research team of two U.S. academic researchers, two Dominican nurses, one Dominican faculty member, and five community health workers. After we provided training in interviewing and focus group techniques, and everyone had been certified in research ethics, we conducted 12 focus groups, 12 individual interviews, and a program of participation observation. We analyzed the data as a qualitative descriptive study, and shared the findings locally, nationally, and through four publications internationally (Foster et al., 2010; Foster, Hilliard, Chiang, Hall, & Heath, 2010; Foster et al., 2012; Foster et al., 2014). The study was supported financially by the National Institute of Nursing Research in the United States.

SUSTAINABILITY

As a result of the study, many exciting collaborations began between the community and the nurses and other health providers in the country. Because of the hospital's participation in the study, the visibility of a hospital willing to be involved in research brought new opportunities to become a Center for Excellence in Maternal-Child Health, for example.

As a faculty member, I bring nursing students to the Dominican Republic for service learning and cultural immersion—experiences that are valuable for developing cultural humility and reflective practice among the U.S. nurses. Students have become one source of sustainability in the setting, because U.S. university health professions programs are interested in providing global exposure to their students. In turn, students offer service learning to the sites.

However, the local sites need more than the services nursing or health services students provide, no matter how well meaning. In the ADAMES project, an element that sustains ongoing continuity in the absence of the U.S. nurses or nursing students is an interprofessional interchange. The interchange has enabled U.S. or Canadian students to travel to the Dominican Republic, stay with host families, learn Spanish, and volunteer as doulas in the hospital. This aspect of the project has kept the whole enterprise sustainable, because students pay fees for the experience, and the Dominican nurses manage the project. The fees cover reimbursement for homestay expenses and Spanish lessons as well as funds to improve patient care in the hospital. Most of the funds are used to cover the cost of medications that patients cannot afford. Funds have also assisted in locally designed research projects and hospital renovations.

Despite the successes in research, service learning, and cultural exchange, it would be inaccurate to claim that the Associación ADAMES has created significant, long-term changes in the quality of maternity care among the nurses in the hospital. While efforts continue to find funding for ongoing community projects to improve maternal and community health in the Dominican setting, the previous question remains unanswered: *How can nurses and other health providers work together globally to sustain motivation to give good care (care they know how to provide), in the context of great resource constraints?* It is a question that constantly challenges me.

REQUIREMENTS FOR GLOBAL HEALTH WORK

For those interested in global nursing, there are specific skills that are indispensable. Language proficiency, clinical experience, flexibility, and openness to difference are all necessary to work in global health, whatever the context. These skills, however, are necessary but not sufficient. More than skills, there are two attitudes critical to working in global health. The first one is to have real heart for the work. The second is not to be a "helper." The dynamic of "coming to help," is paternalistic, rarely successful, and demeans the hard and determined work of many locals to improve the situation in their own setting. As Lilla Watson, an Australian aboriginal activist, social worker, and educator once said, "If you have come here to help me, you are wasting our time. But if you have come because your liberation is bound up with mine, then let us work together" (J. DeLibertis, personal communication, December 16, 2013). Global nursing is working together, accompanying each other, as we struggle, grow, and change.

NOTES

1. Proyecto ADAMES was named for Sor Juana Adames, a well-respected former Director of Nursing at the hospital.

REFERENCES

Cronenwett, L., Sherwood, G., Barnsteiner, J., Disch, J., Johnson, J., Mitchell, P., & Warren, J. (2007). Quality and safety education for nurses. *Nursing Outlook, 55*(3), 122–131. doi: 10.1016/j.outlook.2007.02.006.

Fogarty International Center. (2013). *Implementation science information and resources*. Retrieved from http://www.fic.nih.gov/researchtopics/pages/implementationscience.aspx

Foster, J. (2009). Cultural humility and the importance of long term relationships in international partnerships. *Journal of Obstetric Gynecological and Neonatal Nursing, 38*(1), 100–107.

Foster, J., Burgos, R., Tejada, C., Caceres, R., Altamonte, A. T., Perez, L. J., . . . Hall, P. (2010). A community-based participatory research approach to explore community perceptions of the quality of maternal-newborn health services in the Dominican Republic. *Midwifery, 26*, 504–511. doi: 10.1016/j.midw.2010.06.001

Foster, J., Chiang, F., Burgos, R., Caceres, R., Tejada, C., Almonte, A., . . . Heath, A. (2012). Community based participatory research and the challenges of qualitative analysis enacted by lay, nurse, and academic researchers. *Research in Nursing & Health, 35*(5), 550–559. doi: 10.1002/nur.21494.

Foster, J., Gossett, S., Burgos, R., Caceres, R., Tejada, C., Dominguez García, L., . . . Perez, L. (2014). Improving maternity care in the Dominican Republic: A pilot study of a community-based participatory research action plan by an international healthcare team. *Journal of Transcultural Nursing* doi: 10.1177/1043659614524252

Foster, J., Hilliard, R., Chiang, F., Hall, P., & Heath, A. (2010). Team process in community-based participatory research on maternity care in the Dominican Republic. *Nursing Inquiry, 17*(4), 1–7.

Foster, J., Regueira, Y., Burgos, R. I., & Sanchez, A. H. (2005). Midwifery curriculum for auxiliary maternity nurses: A case study in the Dominican Republic. *Journal Midwifery Womens Health, 50*(4), e45–e49.

Foster, J., Regueira, Y., & Heath, A. (2006). Decision making by auxiliary nurses to assess postpartum bleeding in a Dominican Republic maternity ward. *Journal of Obstetric, Gynecologic, and Neonatal Nurses, 35*(6), 728–734.

Freire, P. (1971). *The pedagogy of the oppressed*. New York: Herder & Herder.

Gladwin, C. (1989). *Ethnographic decision tree modeling*. Newbury Park, CA: Sage.

Joint Learning Initiative. (2004). *Human resources for health: Overcoming the crisis: Report of the Joint Learning Initiative*. Retrieved from http://www.who.int/hrh/documents/JLi_hrh_report.pdf

Kretzmann, J., & McKnight, J. (1993). *Building communities from the inside out*. Chicago, IL: ACTA Publications.

Lerner, D. (1977). *Where there is no doctor*. Berkeley, CA: Hesperian Foundation.

Viswanathan, M., Ammerman, A., Eng, E., Garlehner, G., Lohr, K. N., Griffith, D., . . . Whitener, L. (2004). Community-based participatory research: Assessing the evidence. *Evidence Report Technology Assessment (Summary)*, (99), 1–8.

18

Mi Camino, Mis Compañeros

My Journey, My Colleagues

KIM L. LARSON

Editor's Note: Kim Larson, like Jenny Foster (Chapter 17), is also a nurse educator who brings to her teaching a wealth of knowledge and practice. Kim describes how she weaves her global interests into her academic life both at home and abroad. She provides creative approaches to offering global experiences to her nursing students. Her research contributes to our knowledge regarding Latino adolescent health. My career intersected with Kim's at one point when we worked together on a project to improve the health of migrant farmworker women and their children, which Kim describes below.

A MIDWEST BEGINNING

I am a Midwesterner by birth and a 4th-generation immigrant. My paternal great-grandparents immigrated to Wisconsin from Denmark and my maternal great-grandparents came to Wisconsin from Ireland. My grandfather changed the spelling of Larsen to Larson (the Swedish version) to "fit in" with the neighbors. My parents, Helen and Warren, met in 1949 when my mother was teaching and my father was selling International Harvester tractors, which took us to the farming community of Prairie du Chien, Wisconsin. Prairie, located on the Mississippi River with a population of 5,911, was the third-oldest city in the state. The history of the town as a Sioux Indian and French trading post is central to the community.

Early in my life, two nurses were prominent in revealing to me the possibilities of nursing. My mother's sister, Shirley, was the only nurse in our family. She seemed to have good clinical sense, at least her first aid skills were frequently put to the test with numerous children, her own and cousins, running around the house. I recall Shirley wearing her whites; dress, stockings and shoes, coming home from the community hospital to change quickly, light up a cigarette, and rush to the Franklin House. That was the 1960s. My aunt and uncle owned the Franklin House, a local tavern, which seemed to always be open. Shirley worked full-time at the hospital and when she was off she would relieve her husband as cook or bartender. It seemed as if she worked all the time, making her a superwoman in my eyes. My mother was closest to this sister, not only in age but in hobbies; golf, bridge, and dancing. I loved going to the Franklin House to play the jukebox and watch mom and Shirley jitterbug. Sadly, tavern life had a harmful effect on my aunt and uncle; they both died prematurely. The influence of the environment on addictions, like alcohol and tobacco use, made an early impression on me.

The second nurse is one who "showed me the ropes." During high school I worked with Connie Lucas as a nursing assistant in Prairie's community hospital. I was fascinated by the genuine compassion with which she approached each patient and provided care. Her smile and laughter was comforting, and her tales of camping and canoeing on the Mississippi River inspiring to me. My father had died in the same hospital when I was 4 years old, which may be partly why she took a special interest in developing my career interests. I accompanied her whenever she started or discontinued an IV, changed a dressing, or did any number of nursing procedures. I looked forward to going to work every afternoon throughout my high school years. I now find it interesting to reflect on how this community hospital, a place of both loss and growth, helped solidify my career path.

A BROADER VIEW OF THE WORLD

The majority of people around me were of White northern European descent. So my first glimpse of diversity was in my high school Spanish class when Señorita Margarita loaded her students into a van and drove across the state to the great city of Milwaukee. During these field trips, we were placed in Spanish-speaking neighborhoods to order food, ask for directions, and in general, develop another perspective. My reading and writing skills were much stronger than my speaking skills, but I left high school thinking that the ability to speak Spanish was both exotic and practical. Later, my clinical rotations were at hospitals associated with the Mayo Clinic in Rochester, Minnesota, where people from all over the world sought care. Spanish fluency for health care providers was important even in Minnesota in the 1970s.

While I was in the nursing program, my oldest sister, Kate, became a U.S. Peace Corps volunteer in Sierra Leone, West Africa. Travel to Africa during that time was much less common than it is today and communication across continents more limited. Where my sister was excited at the opportunity, I was frightened and sad to be separated by the distance and uncertainty. My mother took all this in and started making plans for us to visit her in Sierra Leone the following year. When we arrived in the village of Kayima, where Kate lived, we heard children calling her, "Sia Kayima," which meant "first sister." It was clear that she had become a part of her African community. After meeting her African friends, I was convinced she was in a place that cared for her deeply.

While I was there, though, I became sick with a gastrointestinal (GI) infection. When the symptoms became severe and I was too weak to walk, I was taken to a hospital that treated the employees of the diamond mines. I remember being in a private room that was clean and comfortable. Once I was able to drink liquids I was able to appreciate the special care I had received. Later, my sister Kate told me how very sick I had been. When I was discharged I spent a few more days recovering at a local missionary compound. The cost of all this is unknown to my family. We never saw a bill. I believe the generosity and compassion we were shown by nurses, doctors, and missionaries in Africa was a life-changing experience that inspired my own cultural journey.

PEACE CORPS: *"THE TOUGHEST JOB YOU'LL EVER LOVE"*

I graduated with a BSN in 1977 and before too long I also became a Peace Corps volunteer. After 3 months of intensive language training and cultural education in Tegucigalpa, Honduras, I left to work in a small hospital in a village in the district of Olancho, located on the Nicaraguan border. The U.S. government provided volunteers with a stipend for living expenses, which was $200 per month. With that amount I was able to rent a house with electricity, running water, and a flush toilet; purchase bottled water; buy food; and save. Like most volunteers, I employed a young woman to wash my clothes in the river. It is hard to believe now that I could save part of my monthly stipend and have someone wash my clothes. My stipend, $2,400/year, placed me among the middle class in Honduras.

The philosophy of the Peace Corps involves matching the expertise of a volunteer (in my case, a U.S. nurse) with the expertise of a host country national (a Honduran nurse). A kind of co-learning was expected to take place. Speaking Spanish was essential to do the job and we had to pass a language competency exam before moving to our village. Deysi and I worked together for 2 years with the goal of building the capacity of the *auxiliaries de enfermeria* (nursing assistants) who were the backbone of the health care workforce in that country. They were responsible for everything from medication administration to newborn deliveries. I always described my job as that of infection control. Deysi and I tried to apply principles of asepsis in an environment with limited resources. We supervised and assisted with cleaning and sterilizing equipment, including disposable items such as gloves, syringes, and needles for reuse. We ensured that beds and floors were disinfected between patients, though often there were two patients to one bed, especially in the maternity ward. All linens were washed by a cadre of women whose sole purpose was to wash and dry these linens by hand. When the clothes lines were full, the rest of the linens dried on the grass outside the hospital. There were days during the rainy season that we did not have clean, dry linens and patients either brought their own or lay on bare mattresses.

I brought my medical–surgical textbook as a guide to nursing care, but what I found more useful was Werner's (1973) *Donde No Hay Doctor/Where there is no doctor*. Hospitals in Honduras were a place where families came as a last resort, after all home remedies failed. For the subsistence farmers in Honduras, even minimal hospital costs were out of reach. The children's ward was always at capacity with dehydrated and malnourished infants and toddlers. Most of the children were too weak to eat and required IV fluids. Contaminated water and a lack of resources to disinfect water were the culprits of so much sickness. Among the newborns, the GI infections were caused by the use of powdered milk formula. At the time, commercial companies were distributing inexpensive and often free powdered milk formula throughout developing countries to accustom women to using formula instead of breastfeeding. Thousands of infants died from mixing contaminated water with the powdered formula.

Protein-calorie deficiency was apparent by the swollen bellies and thin legs and arms of the toddlers and older children. A lack of food weakened the immune system of children, leaving them vulnerable to all kinds of infections, especially respiratory. We encouraged family members to stay and feed their child because there was not enough staff to provide the needed individual attention. Some parents could and others could not. I recall one little boy who stayed at the hospital for a month, finally recovering from severe malnutrition and pneumonia, only to wait another month before his parents were able to return. After his recovery, he would sit up in his crib and smile and giggle at anyone who stopped to chat. I marveled at how a toddler could be so happy without a parent at his side. It was hard to know the residual effect of acute malnutrition on brain development and I never knew if his cheerfulness was a developmental impairment or an appreciation that his basic needs were being met. Either way, most of us began our day by greeting Jose and we felt a huge loss when he eventually went home with his parents.

Adult males were admitted with machete wounds through the one-room *sala de emergencia*. Olancho had a primarily agriculture economy and farmers used machetes as an all-purpose tool. The large, sharp knives could become unwieldy, slip, and result in deep lacerations to digits and limbs. These injuries often required surgical repair, with post-op treatment and wound management. Infections were always anticipated. Alcohol also played a part in some machete injuries. Alcohol was inexpensive and widely available, especially during celebrations and holidays. During *Semana Santa*, Easter Week, a particular fermented liquid was extracted from palm trees, which was known as palm wine. It was drunk through a thin bamboo straw covered at one end with horsehair to filter extraneous materials such as insects or tree bark. This wine, along with *guaro* (sugar cane liquor) and *cerveza* (beer), when drunk in excess caused unruly and dangerous behavior. The Olancho district of Honduras had large cattle ranches and horseback was a common mode of transportation. The region had a reputation of the "wild west." Men would ride into town, drink too much, get into an argument, and brandish a machete or gun. The machete wounds, sometimes fatal, were often due to financial or family disputes after consumption of too much alcohol. The solution at the time was to let "families work it out."

All Honduran physicians were required to complete one year of social service in a rural area of the country as part of their medical school education. This is how our hospital was staffed. Honduran physicians completed their year and left to set up a practice in one of the larger cities. Dozens of physicians came through our community hospital during my 2 years and no one got to know them very well. During this time the neighboring republic of Nicaragua was involved in a civil war that pitted the Sandinista popular movement against then President Somosa (known for human rights violations). Two Nicaraguan physicians, a husband and wife, crossed the Honduran border to our village because, as pro-Sandinistas, their lives were in danger. Hondurans were sympathetic to the Sandinista movement and the hospital administrator gave the doctors refuge and they in turn joined our hospital staff. It was not until I returned to the United States in 1979 that the controversial relationship between the U.S. government and the Somosa regime was revealed.

One of my best friends in the Peace Corps, Chris Garrison, years later became my husband and greatest supporter of my frequent trips back to Central America. His job in the Peace Corps was management of the pine and mahogany forests in the remote region of La Mosquitia. The area was accessible only by small planes that could land on a short, gravel runway. There was no running water, electricity, or flush toilets where he lived. His diet was primarily rice, beans, and tortillas, and on occasion an iguana or tepesquintle (brown rodent in the agouti family). The American Ambassador to Honduras, Mari-Luci Jaramillo, visited Chris and was so impressed with his tenacity and willingness to work in La Mosquitia that she included him in her biography (Jaramillo, 2002). He is the kind of person who warrants inclusion in someone's biography.

So many of the health problems I saw were preventable. The days when I thought I was most helpful were during the country's mass vaccination campaigns when all available nurses and nursing assistants in our village would climb into pick-up trucks with coolers filled with dry ice, vaccines, and supplies. The pick-up trucks would drop us in different villages and we would walk from house to house, cooler in hand, and administer childhood immunizations. Throughout my 2 years as a Peace Corps volunteer, I learned about health care delivery in a developing country and the sense of fatalism among people living without basic necessities. During those years, I wondered if my Peace Corps stipend would have had a greater public health effect if it had financed a water filtration system or well for the village. The Peace Corps slogan, "The toughest job you'll ever love," was tough mostly because I felt like I was doing so little in a place where the need was so great.

PUBLIC HEALTH

The Peace Corps health sector manager, a nurse, steered my nursing education toward the field of public health. I applied to the University of North Carolina (UNC), School of Public Health. One of my projects in the public health program was to work with the director of a federally funded migrant health center located an hour away from the university. At the time, the migrant health center was beginning to serve a growing Haitian population who had migrated from a country where tuberculosis (TB) was endemic. The director needed a graduate student to conduct a review of the literature and determine best practices in the prevention and management of TB, taking into consideration the transient nature of migrant farm work. Expertise and resources for TB care resided with state and local health departments. The importance of both interagency and interstate collaboration with a mobile population was critical for TB care. The migrant health center was fortunate to have Haitian–Creole and Spanish interpreters, services the local health departments needed for adequate follow-up and case management. To a novice public health professional, collaboration seemed like a win-win situation. I learned that systems-level change requires a lot of good faith, trust, and open boundaries that can take years to foster. It was eye-opening for me to observe the partnering agencies become more aware of their respective expertise and to begin to open the door to each other.

Special Projects of Regional and National Significance

After completing a masters in Public Health Nursing, contacts at UNC led me to apply for a position as a maternal child health project coordinator for a special project of regional and national significance (SPRANS) grant (1984–1990). Dr. Elizabeth Watkins, a team of researchers from the UNC School of Public Health, and the director of the migrant health center received funding from the Maternal and Child Health Bureau, U.S. Department of Health and Human Services, to improve the health outcomes of migrant farm worker women and children (Watkins, Larson, Harlan, & Young, 1990). A bilingual multidisciplinary team, including project coordinator, health educator, social worker, nutritionist, and data manager, was located on site at the migrant health center to work with administration, staff, and farm workers. The dominant farm worker subgroups were Latino, Haitian,

White, and Black American. The overall aims of the grant were to assess the health and social needs of migrant women and children, improve interagency and interstate collaboration, and implement effective public health interventions.

One of the public health interventions implemented by the SPRANS grant was an innovative program that trained migrant women as *promotoras de salud*, lay health advisors (LHA). For this program, we looked for women who were already natural helpers in the migrant community. Chris Harlan, a nurse who is trilingual in English, Spanish, and Haitian-Creole, was responsible for the coordination of the LHA program. The complexity of the program cannot be underestimated. First, farm worker women were recruited from each of the three dominant language groups. To find natural helpers we spoke with staff at agencies who worked with farm workers, such as Migrant Head Start and Farmworker Legal Services. Next, health information sessions were organized and delivered in three languages by facilitators with expertise in each language and topic. Chris and Edwin, her husband from Haiti, together found Haitian-Creole and Spanish-speaking health professionals throughout North Carolina willing to volunteer to serve as trainers.

Well child and women's health practices, and healthy eating were the major topics as well as sessions on intimate partner violence and access to community resources. We used Werner and Bower's (1982) *Helping Health Workers Learn* for practical, hands-on activities for teaching health concepts to diverse populations. Over the course of the project, we found that the LHAs shared this information with their peers and that the program effectively strengthened existing migrant networks (Watkins et al., 1994).

Two of the women who completed the LHA program stand out in my memory for their dedication and commitment to the migrant community. Yolanda was a Latina woman from Mexico and Sharon was a Black American woman from Florida. They didn't know each other but they had much in common. As teenagers they worked with their parents in the fields, but they both were determined to complete their education and find opportunities outside of farm work. They had large extended families with whom they traveled to North Carolina each summer. Both women had graduated from high school, married young, and had children. After the LHA training, they were the eyes and ears of their migrant community, sharing with us the problems and the solutions. Their fathers did not want them to take permanent jobs in North Carolina because that would mean separating from the rest of the family when they returned to their winter homes. To stay in North Carolina was a major decision for these women and we believe the LHA training gave them the self-confidence to convince their families that this was an opportunity for their entire family. They both eventually went to college and were employed by the local migrant health center. In retrospect, this project was my introduction to community-based participatory research.

While working on the SPRANS grant, I received a World Health Organization fellowship to study the health beliefs and practices of areas in Mexico where a majority of the Latino farm workers originated (Larson, 1988). I spent a month in the southern states of Guerrero, Oaxaca, and Chiapas and studied under official public health workers as well as traditional healers. While there I was given a book, which was hand-written and illustrated by one of the traditional healers, of all the local plants, fruits, and vegetables with their identified medicinal properties. I have used this book as both a reference when I worked with migrant farm workers and in the courses I teach with nursing students.

NURSING EDUCATION

I soon found that nursing education provided an opportunity to merge my interests in cultural diversity with public health nursing practice and took a nursing faculty position at a small liberal arts college in eastern North Carolina. One of my colleagues had developed a summer independent study course with the Cherokee nation in the western part of the state. I adapted that course for nursing students who wanted experience with migrant farm workers at the local migrant health clinic. The course offered students an opportunity to learn about the migrant health system, participate in health care delivery in the clinic and outreach to the migrant labor camps, and develop cultural sensitivity. These students often remarked that although they had lived in the area all their lives, they did not know of the health and social issues facing migrant farm workers.

Study Abroad Program: Honduras

The college was affiliated with the Disciples of Christ Church, and the Global Ministries Office of the Disciples of Christ had a working relationship with the Christian Commission for Development (CCD) in Honduras. The CCD was an interdenominational Honduran-led organization that provided aid and technical assistance to rural communities in Honduras. In 1996, the college chaplain and I took students from nursing and religious studies programs to Honduras to work with CCD. During the 2 weeks we completed an assigned construction project and made visits to cultural centers such as El Tigre, the national rain forest, and the Mayan ruins in Copan. Most evenings, Honduran experts in history, anthropology, and education from the local university came to speak with students.

We also spent several days in the village where I worked as a Peace Corps nurse. I had no telephone numbers in which to notify someone in advance of our arrival, and Internet was not yet available in remote areas of developing countries as it is today. During the 3-hour bus ride from Tegucigalpa to Juticalpa I was concerned that no one would remember me and the whole trip would be a bust. I could not have been more mistaken. I was told where the new public hospital and clinics were located, constructed in partnership with the Japanese government. A nursing assistant and I recognized each other immediately and Concepcion asked, "Where have you been?" as if I left yesterday and not 20 years ago. She led me to the director of nursing, a former nursing assistant who had since received her university nursing degree. Maria Elena took me straight to the laundry to demonstrate the automatic washers and dryers, then to the kitchen to show me the stainless steel appliances, and finally to the Chief Medical Officer to receive approval for the nursing students to observe in the hospital. The next couple of days nursing students observed in labor and delivery, emergency, pediatric care, and various clinics. The neonatal unit with seven incubators was one of the most impressive features of the new hospital center.

Study Abroad Program: Peru

The second study abroad program I conducted was in Peru. A Peruvian–American student in our nursing program had family members in Peru who assisted us with travel and lodging. In 1999, seven nursing students and I spent 2 weeks in and around Lima and Cuzco learning about several international health care organizations. One organization, the Heifer Project International, had both a guinea pig project and a red worm composting project. We observed how these projects provide a sustainable food source for the lowest-income communities. To this day, I include the Heifer Project International in my community health course and find it remarkable that so few students have heard of it. It's been gratifying to hear from many former students about the many water buffalo, goats, and guinea pigs they have purchased.

Another organization we spent time with was Partners in Health (PIH), the nongovernmental organization established by Dr. Paul Farmer. Peruvian public health nurses working for PIH took us on home visits to individuals who had recently recovered from TB. One young woman we visited explained how she nearly died because the local health department only had the standard TB treatment. Her TB was multi-drug resistant. She said she owed her life to PIH because they gave her the right medication. During our visit she brought out a small bottle of champagne and poured a shot glass for each of us to celebrate her recovery.

NURSING RESEARCH

Three nurses and one anthropologist played strategic roles in my path to the PhD in nursing. The dean of the nursing program at the college where I taught had a vision of eastern North Carolina where nurses were culturally sensitive and had a global understanding of health care. She took an interest in my career development and encouraged finding a research program that built on my experience with Latino populations. I began the doctoral program at the UNC-Chapel Hill School of Nursing in the fall of 2000. This was at a time when the U.S. census reported that North Carolina was one of three states in the nation that experienced the greatest increase in Latino population growth.

Chris McQuiston, the only nursing faculty in the School of Nursing working with Latino populations, had an NIH project to design community-based interventions related to HIV/AIDS prevention strategies. My familiarity with lay health advisors facilitated my involvement with one component of her research, the *Protegiendo Nuestra Comunidad* program. This program trained natural helpers in an urban Latino community to provide information and support to community members for the prevention of HIV/AIDS (McQuiston, Larson, Parrado, & Flaskerud, 2002). At her recommendation I read the works of Paulo Freire (1970) on popular education and Meredith Minkler (1999) on community building for health.

The following summer I conducted a pilot study with Latino boys and girls in rural eastern North Carolina, which explored the general health concerns of adolescents (Larson & McQuiston, 2008). One of the major findings from the pilot study was that young Latina girls, average age 12 years, spoke about unwanted sexual advances by males. Prior studies had found that Latina girls were at sexual risk at younger ages than adolescents in other ethnic groups. This pilot study led to my ethnographic study of sexual risk among Latino adolescents in eastern North Carolina (Larson, 2009).

Entrée in the Field

Gaining trust and acceptance is an important part of research with Latino families. As a member of the community where I conducted my research, I had participated in numerous community-based initiatives with Latino families including outreach clinics, Sunday school classes, and farm worker festivals. As a bilingual nurse I had worked with Latino adolescents and their parents in migrant health clinics, health departments, and school-based health centers. This foundation, including my Peace Corps experience, facilitated my entrée in the field. At the same time, I was a mother of a teenage daughter. The course work in the doctoral program, my experience in school-based health centers, and my own daughter's transition into adolescence brought a new understanding of the complex issues facing all adolescents in this country. These complex issues, when combined with migration, gender, and cultural norms, had the potential to heighten the vulnerability of Latino adolescents.

Ethnography and Nursing Research

I used an ethnographic approach to guide my participant observation in a selected school and the surrounding community. I also conducted in-depth interviews with a total of 56 Latino adolescents, their parents, and teachers (Larson, 2009). I spent one year in the field collecting these data, immersed in the Latino culture of eastern North Carolina. I observed classroom teaching, made home visits, and upon invitation I attended events important to the Latino community. I was invited to the *fiesta de los quince años*, the 15th-birthday celebration of numerous participants in the study. Interviews with participants and community events highlighted the importance of this cultural rite of passage, yet I was told that some girls were denied their *fiesta*. I found that for most families in this study, the cultural rite was protective of a young girl's sexuality and therefore had a role in the management of sexual risk. However, the social context of the school and community facilitated deviations from traditional norms. Contextual factors included a school environment that provided opportunities for engaging in sexual risk behaviors, caused impediments to sex education, and left teachers confused about cultural norms and stereotypes (Larson, Sandelowski, & McQuiston, 2012). Both teachers and Latino parents were reluctant sex educators.

During data analysis, I became aware of an award-winning documentary titled, *La Quinceñera* (Clements, Glatzer, & Westmoreland, 2006), and a major work of non-fiction (Alvarez, 2007) that juxtaposed sexual risk behaviors and teenage pregnancy with the *fiesta de los quince años*. My study suggested that migration and separation of family networks may weaken the protective mechanism of this cultural rite of passage and that early adolescence (age 11 or 12 years) may be an appropriate starting point for initiating sexual health dialogue between parents, adolescents, and health professionals. This was at a time when the public schools of North Carolina had an abstinence-only sex education policy. It was years later that parents in the state advocated for comprehensive sexual health education and the legislature passed the Healthy Youth Act of 2009.

COMMUNITY ENGAGEMENT

After completing my doctoral program, I took a nursing faculty position at East Carolina University (ECU) in Greenville, NC. The College of Nursing was a designated National League for Nursing Center of Excellence and the University was classified as an "Engaged University" by the Carnegie Foundation. This meant that the University and College of Nursing had a commitment to community engagement. Eastern North Carolina had been my home since 1993 and I saw a real opportunity to further my interests in nursing education while continuing to work collaboratively with the Latino community at home and abroad.

Guatemala

When I joined the faculty, the College of Nursing did not have a study abroad program for undergraduate nursing students. Based on my previous work in Honduras and Peru and a colleague's experience in Guatemala, we developed a global nursing course with language acquisition and service learning as foundational components.

We developed a partnership with *La Unión Centro Lingüistico,* a language school and community development organization in Guatemala. The director of *La Unión* had previously worked for the U.S. Peace Corps in Guatemala and modeled the language school and community development after Peace Corps principles. *La Unión* provides educational scholarships for Mayan children and develops linkages for needed community service work.

Our first study abroad program was designed to include preexperience and postexperience seminars on campus and 3 weeks of cultural immersion in Guatemala. During the campus seminars students and faculty discussed historical, socioeconomic, and ethical issues related to health from faculty in anthropology, bioethics, and nursing. Readings facilitated discussion about immigration and Spanish language skills (Nazario, 2006). The relevance and importance of reflective journal writing was also emphasized.

While in Guatemala, students took Spanish lessons every morning with an individual Guatemalan teacher. In this way, lessons were tailored to the student's language level and interest. Students lived with a Guatemalan family, participated in family and community events, and helped with family chores. Community service proj ects included informal health talks with public school children and mothers' groups. Nursing students developed creative teaching methods, such as interactive games, songs, and sociodramas, to deliver the health information. The students also volunteered in a residential nutrition center for undernourished children and a hospital for the physically disabled.

Each year we assisted a Guatemalan physician with a primary care outreach clinic in the village where *La Unión* had several community development projects. At the outreach clinic we primarily saw mothers and children for two main problems: GI illness—often affecting an entire family and respiratory infections, swollen tonsils, bronchitis, or pneumonia. As I learned in Honduras, these problems can be prevented with clean water and improved cook stove ventilation. This mountain village has difficulty with access to clean water, relying on a small spring and rainwater for drinking. The students and I set a goal with community members to provide every family with a water filtration system. We partnered with *Soluciones Communitarias,* a nonprofit organization in Guatemala to deliver, instruct on, and install over 80 filtration systems.

Following participation in the immersion program in Guatemala, students are placed in a community health setting in eastern North Carolina that serves a Latino population. The students continue to speak

Spanish and apply the cultural knowledge they have learned. One year students who went to Guatemala generated such interest among their peers that safe drinking water became the nursing class gift. The class raised $5,000 for a well to be dug in a Guatemalan community.

Eastern North Carolina

I began my work with the founder of the Hispanic Community Development Center of Wayne County following a series of coalition-building meetings on Latino child health. A natural partnership developed as a result of our joint work on the coalition and a mutual interest in improving the health of the Latino community. At his invitation, I began attending monthly board meetings, got to know other Latino leaders, and assisted with events in the Latino community. I spent a year participating extensively in Center-sponsored events and learning from board members. Part of my contribution at the board meetings was sharing current public health reports regarding the Latino population. These reports routinely highlighted health disparities and health inequalities.

The Center had a small budget that came from industry support (employers of Latino workers) and members wanted to grow the organization. The first grant award we received was from Hispanics in Philanthropy, Inc., an international collaborative that provides planning and implementation grants to Latino-led nonprofit organizations. The aims were to build an active and responsive board of directors, establish an on-site computer resource center, and strengthen partnerships between the Center and mainstream organizations. A second grant followed for HIV/AIDS prevention training for board members. A third grant built on the first two and established the Center as a non-traditional test site for HIV/AIDS.

Over a 4-year period, board members and I collaborated on population need identification, program design, and implementation activities. Perhaps one of the greatest achievements was that an authentic partnership was established between Latino leaders and university representatives. Through leadership training, board members increased their competence with research skills in data collection and protection of human participants, and community development skills in grant-writing and program planning. I learned about the financial struggles of a small community-based nonprofit advocacy group and the dynamic nature of board membership. The Center reaped benefits from the establishment of linkages with mainstream organizations, such as the Area Health Education Center (AHEC), Community College, and the Health Department. The community college expanded English as a second language classes provided on site at the Center. Several Board members completed the certification course for medical interpreters offered through the AHEC, while another was appointed to the local board of health. One board member began coursework to apply to a nursing program. Moreover, they believed in their role to curb the rise of HIV in the Latino community and took pride in establishing the first Latino-led HIV nontraditional test site in the state.

Testing the Feasibility of *¡Cuídate!*

Sexually transmitted infections and teenage pregnancy are still disproportionately higher in the Latino population in North Carolina. Eastern North Carolina is characterized by high poverty rates, lack of access to care, and a conservative view of social issues. Geography plays a large part in sexual health disparities. In fact, North Carolina has been identified as a key state needing sexual risk reduction interventions designed specifically for Latino youth (Cardoza, Documet, Fryer, Gold, & Butler, 2012).

The General Assembly of the North Carolina Legislature passed the Healthy Youth Act in 2009, which mandated the provision of comprehensive reproductive health and safety education in public schools. This law removed the abstinence-only curriculum that had dominated North Carolina public schools for over a decade and opened up opportunities to use evidence-based practice models to address adolescent sexual health. *¡Cuídate! –Take Care of Yourself* is a culturally designed, evidence-based sexual risk reduction program for Latino youth that is supported by the Centers for Disease Control and Prevention (Villarruel, Jemmott, & Jemmott, 2012). This program was first tested with Puerto Rican adolescents in Philadelphia and found to reduce sexual activity, number of sexual partners, and unprotected sex, and increase condom use (Alvarez, Villarruel, Zhou, & Gallegos, 2010).

We tested the feasibility of *¡Cuídate!* in a pilot study with adolescents of Mexican and Central American heritage in rural eastern North Carolina, using a community-based participatory research model. Our research team included faculty from the ECU College of Nursing and College of Human Ecology, school nurses, and a former board member of the Hispanic Community Development Center. All team members were trained in the *¡Cuídate!* curriculum and in the protection of human participants in research.

The pilot was conducted in 2013 in two school-based health centers serving the largest Latino population (>30%) in the county. Following appropriate institutional review board (IRB) protocols, 10 males and 10 females participated in *¡Cuídate!* the sexual risk reduction program. Program modules were highly interactive, with friendly team competitions in games such as *La Zona Peligrosa*/The Danger Zone, where teams competed to correctly identify the risk level for a variety of sexual and nonsexual behaviors. Activities, such as *La Loteria*/Bingo and the safer sex jeopardy game, provided an interactive review of content. Participants engaged in role-plays and were evaluated by other participants using the S.T.O.P. technique (SAY no to unsafe behavior, TALK it out, OFFER explanations, and PROVIDE alternatives).

We collected both process and outcome measures and found that intention to use condoms and knowledge of HIV/AIDS was increased in this pilot group. The program provided a forum for discussing sexual health in the context of cultural norms and family values. It was highly rated by the participants, especially the mixed gender groups and the condom skills-building module. This program was a radical intervention for public schools in eastern North Carolina because comprehensive sexuality education had not yet been fully implemented. This program was unique in that for the first time in this region school nurses and Latina community members were full members of a research team. Still, the success of the program has been the result of years of preliminary groundwork, relationship-building, and cultural understanding with Latino communities locally and internationally.

EL FUTURO

My journey toward cultural understanding has spanned more than 35 years and is a result of friends and family members who sparked my interest and encouraged my passion. Their counsel and friendship made the road I traveled possible. When I think of the future, I think of the roles that education, research, and practice will play in global health nursing.

I am convinced that language skills will give nurses greater credibility when working with Latino communities. Nurses who have these skills are better prepared to understand the needs of the population and deliver culturally relevant services and programs. This means that public schools and universities need to make second languages a priority for both personal and professional development. Since Spanish is the language spoken by the majority of the world's population, it is advantageous that U.S. students acquire this skill.

Nursing education needs to establish mentoring programs that develop faculty in global health nursing. I coteach the study abroad program in Guatemala with a colleague 15 years my junior. Her expertise in leadership and mental health and mine offer students broader perspectives that make this course more interesting. Other venues to keep global health nursing viable would be to establish an active Global Health Committee in a nursing program and develop a global health goal in the strategic plan, as we have done at our college of nursing.

Like other researchers, we recommend widespread application of community-based participatory research (CBPR) when working with the Latino community. In these communities, assets are often unrecognized and organizational power can easily dominate the local "voice." Investing in the CBPR approach will build on community assets and resources, and strengthen existing social networks. A comprehensive handbook is available that clearly provides the essential steps for communities and universities to be successful in CBPR (Israel, Eng, Schulz, & Parker, 2013).

More colleges and universities are developing long-term relationships with community-based organizations in communities at home and abroad. Partnerships that are based on trust and shared power, such as those between ECU and *La Unión* and the Hispanic Community Development Center, can be mutually beneficial for the community and the university. I have found the Latino community in Guatemala and North Carolina to be engaged and invested in their respective futures. I hope to continue to participate in improving the health of Latino families and communities for years to come.

REFERENCES

Alvarez, J. (2007). *Once upon a quinceañera*. London, UK: Penguin.

Alvarez, C., Villarruel, A. M., Zhou, Y., & Gallegos, E. (2010). Predictors of condom use among Mexican adolescents. *Research and Theory for Nursing Practice: An International Journal*, 24(3), 187–196.

Cardoza, V. J., Documet, P. I., Fryer, C. S., Gold, M. A., & Butler, J. (2012). Sexual health behavior interventions for U.S. Latino adolescents: A systematic review of the literature. *Journal of Pediatric Adolescent Gynecology*, *25*(2), 136–149.

Clements, A., Glatzer, R., & Westmoreland, W. (2006). *Quinceañera [Motion picture]*. Culver City, CA United States: Sony Pictures Classics.

Freire, P. (1970). *Pedagogy of the oppressed*. New York, NY: Herder and Herder.

Israel, B. A., Eng, E., Schulz, A. J., & Parker, E. A. (Eds.). (2013). *Methods for community-based participatory research for health*. San Francisco, CA: Jossey-Bass.

Jaramillo, M-L. (2002). *Madame Ambassador, The shoemaker's daughter*. Tempe, AZ: Bilingual Press/Editorial Bilingüe.

Larson, K. (1988). Enhancing migrant health programs: A cross-cultural approach. *Studies & Papers, VI*, 41–47.

Larson, K. (2009). An ethnographic study of sexual risk among Latino adolescents in North Carolina. *Hispanic Health Care International, 7*(3), 160–169.

Larson, K., & McQuiston, C. (2008). Walking out of one culture into another: Health concerns of early adolescent Latinos. *Journal of School Health, 24* (2), 88–94.

Larson, K., Sandelowski, M., & McQuiston, C. (2012). "It's a touchy subject": Latino adolescent sexual risk behaviors in the school context. *Applied Nursing Research, 25*, 231–238.

McQuiston, C., Larson, K., Parrado, E., & Flaskerud, J. (2002). AIDS knowledge and measurement considerations with unacculturated Latinos. *Western Journal of Nursing Research, 24*(4), 354–372.

Minkler, M. (1999). *Community organizing & community building for health*. New Brunswick, NJ: Rutgers University Press.

Nazario, S. (2006). *Enrique's journey, The story of a boy's dangerous odyssey to reunite with his mother*. New York, NY: Random House.

Villarruel, A. M., Jemmott, L. S., & Jemmott, J. B. (2012). *¡Cuídate! A culturally-based program to reduce sexual risk behavior among Latino youth* (2nd ed). New York, NY: Select Media, Inc.

Watkins, E. L., Harlan, C., Eng, E., Gansky, S. A., Gehan, D., & Larson, K. (1994). Assessing the effectiveness of lay health advisors with migrant farmworkers. *Family and Community Health, 16*(4), 72–87.

Watkins, E. L., Larson, K., Harlan, C., & Young, S. (1990). A model program for providing health services to migrant farmworker women and children. *Public Health Reports, 105*(6), 567–575.

Werner, D. (1973). *Donde no hay doctor/Where there is no doctor*. Palo Alto, CA: Hesperian Foundation.

Werner, D., & Bower, B. (1982). *Helping health workers learn*. Palo Alto, CA: Hesperian Foundation.

19

Do No Harm!

A WHO Nurse Looks Back

JOYCE SMITH

Editor's Note: The role of international consultant is described in great detail by Joyce Smith and Pam McQuide (Chapter 20). Joyce is an Irish nurse who has worked for many years in Asia with the World Health Organization (WHO). She leads us through the process of providing technical assistance to organizations and governments with the admonition: Do no harm!

It has been an amazing year; one that has given me an opportunity to reconnect with many of the people with whom I first embarked upon my nursing career. As I sit in my home in Indonesia, I look back on my youth as a heedless Irish school leaver with no idea of what she wanted to do in life. I reflect on how I ended up as a nurse who is a leading expert in the field of Human Resources for Health, working with countries that are in transition following conflict or political upheaval. It has been a long but wonderful journey and I would not have swapped one moment of it for anything.

BECOMING A NURSE

When I left school in 1970 I didn't know what I wanted to do. Resisting my father's wish for me to be a teacher, I agreed to undertake a secretarial course that allowed me to cruise, while being bored rigid by the subject, spending most afternoons at the cinema! The crunch came when a family friend involved in the early days of Irish television offered me a job as a secretary to a producer—a job most Irish girls would have given their eye teeth to have. However, having not attended class, my shorthand and typing skills were nonexistent. I was cornered. I blithely told my parents that I didn't want to be a secretary (true) but instead wanted to do nursing and that I planned to go to London to train. They were not happy with this new choice of career! The idea of nursing training in England was motivated by a desire to get away from home, have a roof over my head, and my need to have breathing space to decide what I actually wanted to do with my life, which I was sure was not nursing.

I was accepted for training at Westminster hospital in London and found to my amazement that I loved it. I felt I had finally found my path in life. This was my first eureka moment and I did not know then that I would have many more along my career path.

In 1972, after completion of training, I took off with my sister and a nursing colleague on the "hippie trail" to India. It was a wonderful 6-month trip that made me realize that we were just skimming the surface of the countries we passed through. I determined that the next time I traveled I would go to work and live.

Returning from the "hippie trail" with severe Hepatitis A, with its associated tiredness and depression, and physically unable to return to the rigors of hospital nursing, I decided to return to school for Public Health Nursing training, which allowed me a year in college to recover. I began my community nursing career as a Health Visitor in a low-income multicultural area of London. I had my next eureka moment feeling that I had really found my vocation in working with families and communities.

EMBARKING ON INTERNATIONAL WORK

In 1976 I took off to Thailand with an English nongovernmental organization (NGO) as part of a four-person medical team to establish health services in a Laotian refugee camp. While reflecting with one of my nursing colleagues from that time we both agree that our initial motivation was that of "wanting to help," which made us feel good. We thought we were hot shots, all London Teaching hospital-trained professionals. We launched ourselves upon the refugee population to establish a U.K.-type of service. It took us about 6 months—getting to know a little of the language and culture—to begin to realize that perhaps what we had established might not be the most appropriate for the situation. I now ashamedly remember dismissing advice given to me by older internationally experienced health professionals and wish I had had the humility to listen.

I continued working with the same NGO in resettlement programs for Indochinese refugees in the United Kingdom and then moved to Hong Kong with a former Thailand colleague to establish health services in refugee camps. This time being older and wiser we applied the lessons learned. We were far more careful in approaching our task to develop an infrastructure including record systems, supply lines, and referral systems. We already knew how difficult it is to establish a functioning system when you start without one in the first place! We then watched as wonderful, concerned, caring health professionals gave up a month of their leave to join us in what was an internationally publicized emergency. Like we had done years before, they leapt off the plane and started treating patients in the absence of any system. We then watched the ones who remained for a longer period struggle, as we had, to readjust what had been started. Did we advise them? No, only if requested. We remembered that we had been just the same and hadn't wanted to be advised.

After Hong Kong I returned to London and became the first "non-doctor" to enroll in the master's course in International Maternal and Child Health. The opportunity represented an experiment to involve other health professionals. It seemed to have worked, as subsequent courses included other professions. While I struggled with microbiology and immunology, my training as a health visitor put me far ahead of my medical colleagues in such areas as community health, teaching, and psychology.

It was a wonderful course, one which helped me put many of my experiences into context. Daily I found myself thinking, *"If only I had known this,"* or, *"If only I had viewed a situation in this light, I could have been much more effective."* It was also a unique opportunity to fly the flag for nursing.

The course cemented my decision to continue to work internationally. I went to work in Brunei Darussalam, a small oil-rich sultanate on the north coast of Borneo in 1984.

BEING THE RIGHT PERSON IN THE RIGHT PLACE AT THE RIGHT TIME

I accepted the post of Nursing Officer for School Health, mainly because I was running out of money after finishing my studies in London. Flying into Brunei, I kept telling myself that even if the work wasn't very interesting I was going to complete the 3-year contract, though it sounded like a life sentence. To my delight it was a wonderful and interesting place to work, particularly in 1984. Brunei had just become independent, accepted Primary Health Care (PHC) as its official approach to health care, and joined WHO; however, few people actually understood what PHC was. As I had studied under one of the founding fathers of PHC, Professor David Morley, I seized the opportunity to contribute.

Brunei, in common with many oil rich countries, depended upon expatriates for the majority of their senior technical positions. In Public Health there were only two Bruneian Nursing officers, the remainder of the nurses were Assistant Nurses. There was a Registered Nurse (RN) cadre but they mainly worked in hospital. The school nurses I worked with were bright and intelligent. I was really upset that they were stuck at assistant level; they deserved the right to progress.

When the Ministry of Health (MOH) requested a WHO nursing consultant to develop a PHC-focused Public Health Nurse training, I immediately got involved. I was fortunate to work with a wonderful Korean consultant, from whom I learned so much, together with the senior Bruneian Nursing officers. I persuaded my staff to take the course—while urging their husbands to be supportive of their training—which would lift them up from Assistant level.

Simultaneously an initiative was begun within the Ministry of Education to establish a Nursing College linked with a British University. The curriculum was based on the British model; however, it required considerable adaptation to reflect a PHC and Brunei cultural context. Having, at this stage, moved from School Health to set up a PHC Training Centre, both my Bruneian colleague and I worked closely with the college to develop and adapt the community training module and provide more extensive community experience. This included having students spend a week in the interior of the country at a settlement of 3 indigenous tribes, living in the jungle, as we implemented PHC. These urban students, stepping out of their air-conditioned cars, had to sleep on floors, wash in the river, and trek many hours to isolated longhouses. They implemented suitably adapted health education in the local school (performance assessed by the local teacher and the head man); they participated in longitudinal nutrition assessment of the school children and worked with the health volunteers from each longhouse. It was a wonderful time and I learned so much from the local community, as did the students. I was determined that urban nurses would never again look down on rural patients and would tailor their preparation for discharge to the conditions to which their patients returned.

Obviously much has changed in the past 20+ years in Brunei. The nursing profession is strong and they host excellent nursing conferences that have a wide international attendance.

INVITATION TO JOIN THE WORLD HEALTH ORGANIZATION

In 1988 I was very excited to be approached by the WHO office of the Western Pacific Regional Office offering me work in the Kingdom of Tonga, a small Pacific Island nation. The work was to redevelop the old 1960s-style basic RN curriculum into an updated PHC-focused one.

The Tongans are ethnic Polynesians who were experiencing an epidemic of noncommunicable diseases, particularly diabetes, due to changes in their traditional diet. Shockingly, almost 50% of all surgery in the country at that time was related to diabetes. The curriculum, under revision, was an apprenticeship-based 1960s model that was task oriented instead of patient centered and included little public health.

I left Brunei sadly but excitedly. I knew Tonga would be a tough assignment. My experience in Brunei taught me that in small countries interpersonal relations frequently get magnified and cause blockages. Tonga had an even smaller population than Brunei.

It took time to adjust to Polynesian culture, which is very different from South East Asian culture. Islanders appear much more "up front." Conscious that I could lose the game on day one if I upset someone inadvertently, I applied what I now advise newcomers to international work to do:

> Keep your head down, your mouth firmly closed, and your eyes and ears wide open for the first few months until you have got the measure of the situation and the people you have to interact with.

It takes time to get a flavor of the culture and the internal politics before you can very delicately start to move.

In doing so I noticed a lot of similarities with the Irish. Indeed, Tongan life reminded me a lot of the Ireland I had grown up in during the 1950s and 1960s. Taking courage from this revelation, I tentatively tried to handle situations as I would in Ireland, and to my relief it often worked. I was very conscious of the fact that if I upset the senior nurses, any work I did would be rejected by them. I also was rapidly learning that doing international work for an agency such as the WHO did not require purely technical skills; it required diplomacy, cultural sensitivity, and above all a willingness to listen, adapt, and recognize the strengths of your national counterparts. As consultants and specialists we have particular skill sets but our national counterparts have local knowledge of the politics and the conditions that have to be adapted to. We ignore these at our peril.

There is no automatic acceptance or respect for us as "experts." In every country and situation we have to earn respect and acceptance through our own approach and actions. However, a willingness to listen and understand, a spirit of working together in partnership, and essentially letting your national counterparts know that you are "*Batting on their team, NOT batting against them*" goes a long way toward working more effectively within a tight time frame.

The time invested in assessment at the beginning of an assignment is THE single most valuable strategy we can employ. It is essential if you don't want your assignment report, plan, curricula or whatever to end up in the bin after your departure, or more likely to sit gathering dust on a shelf and eventually be fodder for bookworms!

This strategy paid off in Tonga and together we developed a new curriculum that was PHC-focused and included a move to student-based training. The community health module was strengthened to better address the issue of rising noncommunicable disease rates. A family-inclusive nursing process was introduced and students were encouraged to think epidemiologically both on the wards as well as in the community. In Tonga, food is equated with love, and while there was much health education provided to communities it was generally ignored. Families were much more likely to listen when there was a crisis, such as someone having a foot amputated as a result of diabetes. The nurses were trained to make use of this window of opportunity in the hospital to teach the family about why their unhealthy diet caused the problem in the first place.

Nurses were asked to estimate the percentage of patients on a ward being treated for preventable conditions. They then devised strategies to target patients and their families, particularly when families brought unhealthy foods to the patient on the ward.

Another crucial issue was that of addressing the needs of graduates who, having been trained in optimum conditions, are then posted to isolated islands or facilities where equipment and supplies used for their training are unavailable. Inadequate preparation for less-than-optimum conditions is a major contributor to low morale in nurses posted to isolated areas. Therefore, training and assessment of nursing procedures should include their ability to adapt safely under these conditions. In my opinion, not addressing this issue continues to be a weakness in nursing education.

Throughout the process doctors were provided an orientation to the new curriculum, its approach, and expected educational standards. They gradually became great supporters of the new approach.

CAMBODIA—THE STEEPEST LEARNING CURVE OF MY LIFE

In 1992 following the Paris Peace Accord, Cambodia, a country that had experienced more than 25 years of war including almost 5 years of mass genocide under the Khmer Rouge, was moving toward peace and holding its first elections in 25 years. I was in Tonga at the time and implementation of the new nursing curriculum was going apace. Having worked in refugee camps on the Thailand borders in the mid-1970s, I was aware of many of the happenings in Cambodia. I felt a great urge to contribute to the reconstruction of Cambodia. As Cambodia fell under the World Health Organization/Western Pacific Regional Office (WHO/WPRO), for whom I worked, I immediately applied for a transfer. I was granted a transfer that propelled me into what has become my overriding concern: that of redeveloping human resources development systems for Ministries of Health in postconflict and transitional environments.

Nothing in my professional career prepared me for what I faced in Cambodia. Rebuilding a Ministry from the bottom up in a country that had suffered targeted genocide and where there had been a loss of almost a complete generation of role models was the most profound professional challenge. However severe the challenge was for me and my professional colleagues in the WHO, other international agencies, and NGOs, it was even more severe for our national counterparts who had lived through 25 years of war and genocide. Whenever I felt like quitting, I just had to look at my national counterparts in the MOH who, despite having been to hell and back, were finding the strength to rebuild. It was sufficient to make one feel like a wimp and to spur one on again.

I came to Cambodia as the "Training Officer" working as part of the Strengthening Health Systems Project. This reflected the still-prevailing "Personnel and Training Approach" to human resources development (HRD). Arriving in the Ministry I discovered that my role was to redevelop HRD systems, and as my work progressed I discovered that it was much more than personnel and training. Develop human resources (HR) policy from scratch—Help!!—well I had revised policies and plans . . . but do it from scratch . . . Help!!! My constant refrain to myself was . . . "Deep breaths, stay calm, stay practical . . . common sense" before I jumped into the next challenge. I likened it to professional bungee jumping!

One of the first things to be done was to conduct a survey of the entire workforce. Many agencies were trying to do so but they utilized complex forms that were not understood by their national counterparts and consequently did not yield consistent data. When I got my HR team together and explained what we needed, and more importantly why, they had a discussion and came back to me saying that the information we needed could be gathered from payroll records in each province.

I now learned another lesson that has served me well over the years: ask the right questions and explain why we are asking the questions. This approach usually gets you what you need, maybe not 100% of the information you would like to have, but it will get you most of what is essential.

During that time, prior to the first election, the WHO worked with all four political factions to reintegrate what had been separate health systems. The WHO office in Phnom Penh was perceived as a neutral venue where they could come together to discuss technical health issues. A Health Equivalencies Working Group organized by the WHO and United Nations High Commission for Refugees revealed that there were 59 different categories of health workers, of which 17 categories were nurses.

This Working Group—which included representation from all factions—compared training curricula to eventually condense the list down to 22 categories of health workers.

During the war years the Health Professional Training institutions were degraded, as were both primary and secondary education systems. The targeting of educated professionals for genocide meant that the majority of qualified teachers had either died or left the country. To fill the void, top-performing graduates were retained in the schools to teach, barely keeping ahead of the classes they were teaching. The gap between what was known by graduates from secondary education and what was required for entry to tertiary health professional education was very great, particularly in terms of mathematics and sciences. Teachers who trained post-Khmer Rouge in 1979 trained with little clinical experience due to large classes (to try to replace the lost health workers), empty hospitals, lack of books, and equipment. A class of 300 medical students or midwives might have one sphygmomanometer and stethoscope between them all. Most graduated without having witnessed a normal delivery, let alone assisted with one. Training was mostly carried out with only a blackboard and chalk. Teachers taught what they remembered, not what was required for their graduates to do the job. Under these difficult conditions, health professionals who had trained before the war, such as nurses and midwives, were put through emergency training to become medical assistants and doctors, thus depriving the nursing profession of their remaining leaders and role models.

A wonderful Afghan proverb says:

> If you don't know that you don't know you will not reach your destination; if you know that you don't know you will reach your destination.

The first line of this proverb absolutely applied to Cambodia in 1992. International agencies tried to apply Western models of nursing education by recommending that the MOH abandon training of assistant-level nurses. They guaranteed that they would train high-level nurses—equivalent to Western-educated nurses. While this was the ideal, the numbers that could be trained were very small in comparison to what was required. The number of national nurse educators who had sufficient knowledge and skills to teach in these optimal training courses was extremely limited. Graduates of these new training courses did not leave the capital and in fact were mostly employed by private hospitals, resulting in a loss to the government health service, which had trained them. Nor did the graduates go to work in underserved areas. These were the consequences when early in the reconstruction phase the MOH—under pressure from external agencies—embarked on a costly strategy that did not benefit MOH health facilities. Nor did it strengthen the capacity of the large number of assistant nurses who were actually delivering health services to communities to the best of their ability.

One excellent initiative was undertaken by the United Nations Border and Relief Operation (UNBRO). The UNBRO worked with agencies training health workers in the refugee camps on the Thai border to standardize training and set up qualifying examinations to assess the level of knowledge and clinical capacity of the health workers trained over almost 20 years in those camps. This system provided a mechanism so that health workers could be absorbed into the Cambodian workforce appropriately. There had been more than 100 agencies working in health, many implementing their own nonstandardized trainings; some were absolutely excellent. Others, however, were very inadequate—resulting in 59 different categories. The UNBRO Testing and Certification process greatly assisted the MOH of Cambodia. Sadly, I have never found this excellent UNBRO process replicated in other similar postconflict scenarios. Why do we continue to perpetuate flawed approaches yet ignore those that work well?

Another area where "international approaches" caused problems was in getting support to strengthen midwifery training in Cambodia. With the advent of the PHC approach, the training of Traditional Birth Attendants (TBA) was a major strategy. Indeed I had been a great advocate of training for TBAs myself in the 1980s. In Cambodia in the 1990s, despite evidence that TBAs had made little or no significant impact on maternal mortality rates, agencies working in the field of maternal and child health (MCH) continued to fund TBA training without providing support to basic midwifery training. Training programs were implemented by teachers who had trained without clinical practice. Yet the midwifery graduates were expected to take referrals and technically support the TBAs. It took some years to finally obtain support for basic midwifery training.

TBAs have subsequently fallen out of favor internationally and community health workers are back in favor. The world seems to be littered with millions of abandoned TBAs, and I wonder what the next hot item will be. It is this cavalier attitude toward health workers that causes so many HR problems and demoralizes the frontline of least-educated health workers who are expected to carry much of the burden of health care to the most inaccessible populations.

TEACHING AND LEARNING IN THE CAMBODIAN CONTEXT

As it became very clear that teaching skills were weak and needed to be addressed, the WHO permitted me to establish a Diploma in Health Personnel education for teachers of all disciplines from all teaching institutions as well as the specialist centers/institutes (TB, HIV, Malaria, MCH, and public health (PH)). There were 22 participants. At first there was some unease among doctors, dentists, and pharmacists who were university trained about studying with nurses, midwives, laboratory technicians, and physiotherapists—who were not. However, as the course progressed the interprofessional barriers fell as everyone realized they were all struggling with a common subject.

I engaged a very experienced British midwifery educator who had been in Cambodia for 10 years, who spoke and read Khmer, together with a Khmer trainer who had a master degree from Thailand to work with me on its implementation. The course was originally designed to last 9 months but had to be extended to 14 months to allow us to cover all the course content. Efforts to get the course accredited by the University of Phnom Penh failed due to poor relations between the Ministries of Education and Health. However, we were able to obtain support from the University of New South Wales (UNSW) in Australia, which monitored implementation and assessment. While not accrediting the course, because it was not accredited by the University of Phnom Penh, the UNSW was willing to accept graduates for entry in master's degree courses. For the first time, an opportunity was created for nurses, midwives, and allied health professionals who had not trained in degree programs to study abroad.

Implementing this postgraduate course was an exhausting but rewarding experience. Due to the length and depth of the program, we had to confront issues that were often glossed over during short in-service courses. Many of our students grew up during the Khmer Rouge Era as children of war. When the conflict ended, what followed was the emergency approach to training—described earlier—leaving many gaps in their knowledge. As a result of this history, the remaining core group of professionals found it extremely difficult to express opinions, let alone let students do so. To make the situation more difficult, basic equipment, such as surgical gloves, had been unavailable for years and was unknown. How do you teach nosocomial infection control if your target group has never seen something as basic as the gloves being introduced by the aid agencies?

The course was conducted in the Khmer language using a collaborative approach. An excellent NGO who trained trainers for community development introduced the basic principles of training. Course content was then further developed by experts from the Faculty of Education in Phnom Penh University who had studied overseas. My team continued to build on this foundation by encouraging students to apply the principles they had learned to the reality of training health workers.

It took almost 4 months to get across the concept of teaching and learning. We finally had a breakthrough when, over Christmas and New Years, the students were assigned to observe both good and bad teaching in a variety of settings. Several students returned from a prestigious school, telling us:

> "The teachers talked at and told the students, but they didn't TEACH them!"

Needless to say, my teaching team was over the moon! Now we could move on.

Our group of trainee teachers became very motivated, very close, and discussed everything together. In sharing individual breakthroughs they contributed majorly to group understanding.

One of the biggest gaps we discovered was in basic mathematic skills. Prior to commencing the educational assessment module, I administered a basic mathematics test with addition, subtraction, multiplication, and division of regular numbers, decimals, and fractions, for which students were not allowed to use a calculator. They were also given logic problems such as "Province *A* has a population of *x* and has *y* number of doctors, what is the ratio of doctor to population?" Other questions related to calculating mortality rates (given the formula) and calculating drug dosages. There was not one question that all of the 22 students got correct. Only 2 knew what a ratio was and only 5 were able to calculate a crude death rate correctly. There was no difference between professions in Math ability. This result had nothing to do with level of intelligence. For the first time we had evidence of the major impact 25 years of war had on the educational system—including 5 years under the Khmer Rouge when schools were closed, books destroyed, and teachers killed.

This evidence was essential, particularly as many of the technical training courses involved some form of mathematics. Lack of math ability also has an impact on studying the sciences. The presence of digital watches and calculators in many ways concealed the lack of math foundation. We also heard about nurses and other health workers who could not read their watches. And yet, we were introducing training courses that required frontline health workers to time respirations and time pressure cooker sterilization cycles, among other tasks. Providing such evidence to donor agencies contributes greatly to more appropriate use of scarce financial resources and ensures that funding and approaches are more strategically targeted to the individual situation. This prevents replication of blanket, and generally ineffectual, approaches to capacity development.

Happily the gaps in the foundations in mathematics, sciences, and other areas have now been addressed. It is very characteristic of the Cambodians that once they understand "what they do not know" they work exceedingly hard to remedy the situation.

The course continued for a few years supported by another donor, but, because it was not linked to Phnom Penh University, it did not become institutionalized. However, a core of health personnel educators was created and engaged by many agencies working with the MOH.

MOVING ON

I left Cambodia in 1998 after 6 years, completely burnt out and aware that it was time for fresh perspectives from someone else. Because of family commitments I based myself back in Europe. However, I continued short-term work in Human Resources for Health with the WHO at their Regional Office Manila, in Timor Leste from 2000 to 2001, and in Afghanistan in 2002.

Timor Leste, formerly East Timor, had been a Portuguese Colony until 1975. It was then a district of Indonesia before separating from Indonesia in 1999 and gaining independence in 2002.

There had been an ongoing independence struggle. Although the fighting in 1999/2000 was short lived, the majority of the infrastructure was destroyed. Based on experiences such as those in Cambodia, there was an implicit assumption by aid workers that if the physical infrastructure was destroyed, so too was the human capacity. This was not the case in Timor Leste, and the health workforce, trained in the Indonesia health system, remained.

The approach of the majority of aid organizations was "to train" as they had in a post-conflict countries—such as Cambodia—where schools had been destroyed and there had been a massive insult to the numbers and capacity of the health workforce. This caused great frustration and insult to the Timorese health professionals. I well remember, at an HR management workshop at the Dili School of Nursing, an experienced nurse tutor expressing his frustration:

> Who do they [aid agencies] think we are? They come here and tell us about Malaria—this is a mosquito net, this is an anti-malarial drug etc. We are trained professionals living all our lives in a malarial area. We know all about malaria and dealing with it. Do they think we are stupid?

This is a clear example of how, if we start without properly learning about the situation and not listening to and involving our national counterparts, we can get it badly wrong and waste scarce or limited financial and human resource effort. It would have been more appropriate to find out what they knew and identify what updates were required to enhance their knowledge.

On another note, the issues of using and adapting approaches that have worked well appears to be a foreign concept in some situations. Afghanistan, like Cambodia, had experienced 25+ years of war and there had been massive training of health workers in the refugee camps in Pakistan. In 2002, prior to the closing of those camps,

I visited aid organizations in Peshawar who had provided training in the camps. I found that there had been no testing and certification process in the camps, such as had been developed by UNBRO in Thailand. The majority of the agencies had no record of who had been trained in what. This resulted in the MOH having to develop a testing and certification process quickly at a time of redevelopment of the health system, a difficult and politically sensitive task indeed.

The results of the testing and certification process undertaken in 2005 for nurses, midwives, and allied health workers revealed that approximately 50% of people applying to be tested held false certificates. (There was a thriving business in production of false certificates!) Of those who took the exams approximately 25% were actually at the level they claimed. At least 50% required complete retraining. The rest continued to work under supervision and were given three opportunities to retake the examinations over a 5-year period.

These results presented the MOH with a problem: how to fund retraining that had not been anticipated nor budgeted for. Many of the health workers who failed were employed by NGOs that were contracted by the MOH to implement basic health services. The MOH tackled the situation with help from outside agencies that brought in tutors to provide training and coaching to bring staff up to the required standard. Some donor agencies funded production of text books and training materials for those who failed to achieve the required standard. It is to the credit of all involved that the majority of these health workers are now certified.

WHY HUMAN RESOURCES DEVELOPMENT?

While working in Cambodia I realized that human resources are the key factor in successful implementation of any health service. It accounts for up to 80% of any health budget. However, planning, managing, and financing human resources get the least attention of any area in the health system. Having spent more than 20 years working in ministries of health in a number of countries, I am still saddened by the continued highly theoretical, splintered, and uncoordinated approaches to HRD that result in a poorly motivated workforce—the reef upon which beautifully designed health system approaches wreck themselves.

I remember how inadequate and overwhelmed I had felt upon arrival in Cambodia—confronted with the enormity of the task to reestablish an HR system. My background only covered a small part of the whole, and without a guide or access to other people's experiences it was sink or swim. It was the same for my national counterparts who were appointed to posts for which they had little or no experience. In 2005—having had similar experiences in other post-conflict countries and with support from the WHO—I published a "Guide to Health Workforce Redevelopment in Post Conflict Environments." My motivation was not to say "this is how you do it" but to explore and share key issues and questions. It includes examples of what worked where and, more importantly, what didn't work and why.

WORDS OF ADVICE

Life in semi-retirement on my island in Indonesia offers an opportunity to reflect on how the nursing profession is evolving. It is essential to understand that a one-size-fits-all approach will not work in international training. One point stands out. The worldwide trend toward university-based nursing education may not be appropriate in countries where only the wealthy can afford to go to college. Graduates with a high level of education tend to stay in urban areas, as demonstrated in the Cambodian example. Potential students from less urban and rural environments—who are willing to serve isolated communities—have limited access to training. Without an infrastructure to support universal university education, abandoning diploma and assistant level training programs for nurses causes harm to poor and disadvantaged populations throughout the developing world. It is beholden on all of us who work internationally to assess the country situation carefully before acting.

Whether you are starting out for the first time or are an old-timer like me, I wish you well and ask you to remember: "*Keep your head down, your mouth firmly closed, and your eyes and ears wide open for the first few months until you have got the measure of the situation and the people you have to interact with,*" and above all, DO NO HARM!

20

My Life Is an Adventure

It's Not for the Faint Hearted—But It's Worth It!

PAMELA A. McQUIDE

Editor's Note: Pam McQuide has worked for years as an international health consultant—although with NGOs and universities, rather than the WHO, as Joyce Smith (Chapter 19) does. Like Joyce, Pam's insights are practical and affirming and represent best practice in the field of global health consultation. Notice the titles chosen by Joyce and Pam for their chapters. They illustrate the two ends of the spectrum that global health nursing represents!

HOW DID I GET HERE?

First Steps

If you knew me when I was growing up on a small farm in Wisconsin, you would have trouble imagining that one day I would have a doctorate in international health policy and be the country director of an international nongovernment organization living in Namibia. For those growing up in rural Wisconsin it was a milestone to simply complete high school and to get a job. There was no encouragement to go to college. My family claimed only one college graduate. My aunt's husband—who was originally from Austria—used the GI Bill for his education after World War II. Girls were supposed to get married and have kids, not go to university. Somehow that never quite fit my mold. I had a fair amount of innate rebel in me.

I can never remember a time when I was not interested in learning about people from other countries. My Uncle Dutch, mentioned above, ended up being a German language professor at Purdue University even though his wife—my auntie—only finished eighth grade because there were no high schools in the area. I visited them frequently. My uncle allowed me to sit in the library while he taught classes. I dreamed that one day I would go to college. Whenever my uncle traveled on sabbatical my grandmother bought me a couple of international mailgrams so I could write to my aunt and uncle, which I did faithfully.

I had several pen pals, including ones in Thailand, Canada, and England. I didn't know anyone at school who had a pen pal, certainly none with international ones. Another clue about my international interests was when at age 10 I promised our church minister I would become a missionary in Africa. I still remember that conversation and believe that is when I made a true commitment.

Clearly, I did not appear destined for college. After graduating from high school I worked full-time as a secretary for an insurance firm, part-time in a grocery store, and in my dad's office on Saturday mornings. I also started taking evening courses at the local branch of the University of Wisconsin. By the next fall I was enrolled at the University of Wisconsin, Madison. I registered as a French major because I was determined to learn how to speak French. While in college I married a medical student who had recently returned from the Peace Corps in Morocco. He wanted to return to Africa one day and work as a doctor. During that time, I also worked part-time at the hospital, typing up electrocardiogram (ECG) readings for a cardiologist who was paralyzed from the waist down from cancer. He needed someone to push him in his wheelchair to the medical school where he taught medical students how to interpret ECGs. He had a tendency to call on me when the medical students did not know the answers. Although I had never studied biology or chemistry I often came up with the correct response. I started to rethink the French major, realizing that I wanted to do more than speak French. I liked working with people and thought about nursing, but I was scared of the science courses that I had to take with other students that had years of high school science. I decided to enroll in a diploma program so that I could finish by the time my husband completed medical school. Much to my surprise, I actually did better than anticipated, ranking in the upper 90 percentile in most of the sciences! That's how I became a nurse. It was the best decision I ever made.

I loved being a nurse. I think I worked in almost every job nursing has to offer, from nursing assistant to RN over the next 10 years or so. I worked in intensive care, unit teaching, nursing management, and supervision. I loved direct patient care as much as I later enjoyed helping new nurses to become their best professionally. I eventually earned degrees in French and nursing, although my first marriage did not succeed.

Mid-way through my hospital career I became very active in the local branch of the American Nurses Association (ANA). I was particularly interested in how the ANA impacts nursing legislation. In 1986 I attended the Nurse in Washington Internship Program (NIWI), which prepares nurse leaders to become politically active and to impact health policy legislation. One key message I came away with was that "Nurses are this country's sleeping giant we need to wake up. There is nothing we cannot do if we come to the table and stick together." That experience motivated me to chair several legislative committees locally and nationally. I was elected President of the Milwaukee District Nurses Association, through which I taught nurses the importance of impacting health care legislation. Few legislators knew much about health care or even the difference between a nurse practitioner and a licensed practical nurse. In 1 year I gave about 50 talks to schools of nursing and nursing associations. I also invited state policy makers to meet with nurses to better understand health care in Wisconsin.

After making several visits to Washington, DC, and Madison, Wisconsin, to represent the voice of nurses and our patients to policymakers, I left hospital nursing to work as a legislative aide for State Representative Judith Robson, a public health nurse, and chair of the public health committee for the Wisconsin State Legislature. I became involved with crafting legislation such as for expanded immunization coverage for children and direct reimbursement for nurse practitioners for clients on Medicare and Medicaid (before there was a Federal law allowing that to happen). I was particularly touched by the fact that even in a state like Wisconsin, there were many pregnant women with limited or no prenatal care coverage. How could this be?

INTERNATIONAL HEALTH POLICY

For over 20 years I had traveled regularly to France to visit friends. I knew that the French and European health systems, in general, encouraged prenatal care. They mandated that employers allow women paid leave for their prenatal appointments and even gave women financial allowances if they completed the recommended number of prenatal visits. That was not happening in the United States in the early 1990s. My travels to France had a profound impact on my decision to get a PhD in international health policy so I could contribute to improving health services for people in the United States.

I enrolled in the Heller School at Brandeis University to get a PhD in Social Policy. I chose a multidisciplinary program because health policy involves all health professionals, not just nurses. For the first time ever, my (second) husband and I left Wisconsin and moved to Massachusetts. Given the direction my life has taken, I never regretted that decision.

My research interests were centered on maternal and child health (MCH) status in Europe. Although the Heller School was recognized for their policy program, the school did not have strong expertise in international MCH. My professors thought it would be impossible to conduct a study in Europe because they did not have connections with European colleagues. I was not willing to give up. Every paper I wrote in graduate school covered an aspect of European health systems, especially prenatal care. As I completed my coursework and passed my comprehensive exam, I started to seriously think about my dissertation. I ran across a recent edition of the *American Journal of Public Health* and noticed an article comparing systems of prenatal care between the United States, France, Belgium, and Hungary. I wrote to the author, Dr. Pierre Buekens, chair of the MCH Department at the Universite Libre de Bruxelles (ULB), inquiring about access to secondary data so I could compare European systems of prenatal care. A week or so later, as I was sitting at my kitchen table with three colleagues discussing our PhD proposals, the phone rang. It was Dr. Pierre Buekens calling from Brussels to say he had received my letter and "we (ULB) are very excited to hear about your interest in European systems of prenatal care." I learned that the European Union (EU) had just funded a new study called "Barriers and Incentives to Prenatal Care in Europe." The study was designed to examine maternity policies and systems in 17 European countries (including Hungary and Norway, which were not part of the EU in 1995). Dr. Buekens wanted to know if I would be interested in collaborating with the research team for my dissertation and, more specifically, if I would be willing to help them collect the data for Hungary. The rest is history.

Dr. Buekens also had secondary data from a previous prenatal care study in Europe comparing seven countries, but it did not include data from France. I was interested in including France in a secondary data analysis because I knew that the French had the most generous system of prenatal care allowances. Prior to "officially" agreeing that we could work together, I was asked to formally meet with Dr. Buekens at ULB in Brussels. During the meeting, Pierre called a colleague of his in Paris, Beatrice Blondel, at Institut national de la santé et de la recherche médicale (INSERM) (French Institute of Health and Medical Research), equivalent to our National Institutes of Health. Pierre shared with her my interest in participating in the EU study and including secondary data comparisons using French MCH data. He asked Beatrice if she had access to data that could be shared for my study. To this day, I can hear Beatrice loudly exclaim, "An American! What am I going to do with an American?" Pierre kindly replied that I spoke French fluently, I was coming to France the following day, and he would appreciate it if she would be willing to meet with me. Beatrice begrudgingly agreed and I was at INSERM the following day. Fortunately I passed the French test! She agreed to share some of their data if I could work at their INSERM office in Paris. What a hardship to spend time in Paris, especially since I had several friends with whom I could stay! I collected data for Hungary, France, and Belgium for the study. France ended up giving me a "minidatabase" to take home with me.

The lesson I learned from that experience is to never create barriers for yourself just because you don't know how things will work out. This lesson has served me well for many years. It seems that I rarely know how I am going to do something, but I know that it should be possible and I just need to figure out how to do it.

International Maternal and Child Health

Using the data I had collected in France, Belgium, and Hungary for the EU study, I completed my dissertation in May 1997 with the faith that a job would be waiting for me. The day I handed in my final version of the dissertation I returned home and noticed that my answering machine was flashing. A friend had left a message saying that a head-hunter was looking for someone with expertise in international maternal child health and French. So "voila," I accepted a position as

Senior Researcher with Family Health International (FHI) in North Carolina. My title sounds impressive and I was scared. Apart from my dissertation, I had limited experience with research. Now I had to prove that I could do it.

This position allowed me to make my first trip to East Africa, where I eventually conducted an economic study on ability and willingness to pay for family planning services in Kenya. I also made over 20 trips to Haiti to assess quality of family planning services and the effectiveness of various training methods for health workers offering family planning services. In the process I figured out how to conduct qualitative and quantitative research.

Work Force Assessment

My work with FHI positioned me well for a post-doc at Emory University School of Nursing. However, since I ended up conducting a study on prevention of maternal-to-child transmission of HIV/AIDS as a principal investigator (PI), I had to become an assistant professor since post-docs cannot be PIs.

In the long run, the most important aspect of my position at Emory was the evaluation I conducted to determine whether a new degree-level nursing school should be started in Kenya. Although I didn't have much experience in regards to appropriate considerations for starting a new school of nursing, I did know some of the nurse leaders in Kenya, such as the chief nurse and registrar at the Kenyan Nursing Council. It seemed to me that the determination about whether or not a new school was needed should have something to do with current demand for the existing degree-level nurses. So I decided to start by finding out how many diploma nurses and degree-level nurses were in the country and how many were required. This may sound reasonable and simple, but nothing could have been further from the truth. When I asked the chief nurse how many nurses at different levels of preparation were in Kenya, she responded, "I have no idea, but maybe around 25,000." I asked a similar question of the registrar at the Nursing Council (equivalent to the Board of Nursing in the United States) and she replied, "I have no idea, maybe around 50,000. But we don't use the degree-level nurses that we do have."

Instead of going back home defeated, I decided to investigate the inconsistencies in the responses of the chief nurse and the registrar. A review of the data system at the Nursing Council revealed that the council had a separate paper file for each person every time he or she finished a nursing course. Nursing education in Kenya is not offered as a unified curriculum in the way it is in the United States. Over time Kenyan students may be enrolled or be registered in several distinct nursing programs: general nursing, midwifery, community health, as well as in other specialty areas. So one individual could have as many as five or six files for different qualifications earned. Now it made sense why the numbers at first glance seemed so dramatically different. On average each nurse had two separate files at the council, so it appeared that there were twice as many nurses as there were actual individuals. Since all the records were paper based, there was no way to tell how many files existed for the same individual. With this information, I realized we weren't ready to recommend an investment in starting a new school of nursing. Instead, I suggested we conduct a workforce assessment of nurses to identify how many nurses were trained, registered, and licensed to work in Kenya by the different specialty areas. By developing this type of database, I knew that theoretically we could find out how many nurses were trained and qualified in the different specialty areas as well as the unique number of nurses available in the country (under retirement age). This was one of my better decisions professionally, but it also proved to be one of the most challenging. Although I was a researcher, I did not know how to identify someone with the right skill set to develop the kind of database needed. To complicate matters, there was the question of "open-source" or proprietary software code. I had a steep learning curve and made my share of mistakes along the way.

Human Resources for Health Interventions in Africa

Human Resources Information System (HRIS) in Kenya

When I first went to Kenya to assess whether or not they needed a new degree program for nursing, I had no idea it would lead to the development of an HRIS for the Kenyan Nursing Council. After conducting a needs assessment and sharing the results with several key stakeholders in Kenya, they replied, "We have needed this kind of information for so long. Every time I am asked (Registrar, Nursing Council) about how many enrolled and registered nurses I have in Kenya, it takes us weeks to go and count up all of the paper forms (records) we have in storage. I still don't know how many times we are counting the same person. We have 'diplomatitis' where the same person returns to school several times for different nursing qualifications."

Upon my return to Atlanta, the assessment results were shared with the Centers for Disease Control and Prevention (CDC, the funder) and my employer (Emory University) and a decision was made to develop a database that could be kept up to date for the Kenyan Nursing Council. Needless to say, my research background did not prepare me to set up a national database of all nurses, but it did prepare me to know what data fields were required and how to analyze the data once they were available. My learning curve was a straight line ascending high into the clouds. Although I made a variety of errors in selecting a developer and did not initially develop the code in open-source software so we would be given the "source code," a database was eventually produced that could do the kinds of analysis I had initially envisioned.

Perhaps one of the greatest accomplishments with this first fairly rough database was that we were able to share the results with the East Central Southern African Health Ministers' Conference (ECSA) as well as host a special meeting with all ECSA Chief Nurses and Registrars to discuss the importance of nursing data to estimate how many nurses they have and how many are needed to meet the health needs in each country. Because the Kenyan Nursing Council showcased these data for the ECSA Health Ministers, it also put nursing in the forefront to championing the need for better understanding of the supply side for human resources for health information to improve human resources planning, management, policies, and quality of care. During the time I was at Emory, my husband commuted between Atlanta and Raleigh—one of the hazards of a dual-career marriage—so I decided to move back to the Triangle so we could live in the same place.

It was the human resources for health expertise that I seemed to have stumbled upon in Kenya that led me to IntraHealth International when I left Emory and returned to North Carolina. It turned out to be a fortuitous move as IntraHealth International had just been awarded a 5-year global project from USAID called Capacity Project. The aim of the global human resources for health project was to identify requirements for training and deployment as well as improvement of leadership, management, productivity, and retention of health workers, especially in developing countries.

I made an appointment with IntraHealth to see if they needed anyone with my experience in Human Resources for Health (HRH). Much to my amazement, one key activity of the Capacity Project was the development of a Human Resources Information System (HRIS) to track employed health workers. IntraHealth was interested in learning about the current demand for health workers but they hadn't considered the issue of supply of health workers. IntraHealth had recruited a team of brilliant software developers that, however, did not include a clinical person who understood health policy to know what questions these databases should be answering. This is where I stepped in.

For the next 5 years I collaborated with the Capacity Project team working on the HRIS to meet with policy makers in countries such as Rwanda, Uganda, Swaziland, Botswana, Namibia, and Southern Sudan to identify important policy, pre-service training, and management questions. These HRIS databases were developed using "open-source" software so that the code was available to anyone who needed to customize the database to specific country needs. In the end, the HRIS system and results have been shared at multiple international meetings around the world in collaboration with the World Health Organization (WHO), World Bank, and other key international organizations. It was definitely the right time with the right tool, but it also took a village of people with combined skills to make it happen.

Application of the Workload Indicators of Staffing Need (WISN) Tool in Namibia

When I first moved to Namibia as Deputy Chief of Party in September 2011, I actually thought I was the wrong person for the job. The IntraHealth Namibia office dealt with HIV/AIDS-related service delivery and technical assistance and I was an expert in human resources for health. Shortly after arriving I was given the title of Chief of Party (Country Director), a role I had not held previously. However, before long I was sitting on the HRH Technical Working Group (TWG) for the Ministry of Health and Social Services (MoHSS) and asked to help the government figure out how they could effectively absorb all the donor-supported health workers delivering HIV/AIDS related services. At the time most HIV/AIDS-related health workers' salaries were paid for by either the Global Fund or the United States Government. The MoHSS was also in the midst of a restructuring effort since their current staffing norms were over 10 years old and they were not evidence based. I imagine you can now see where this story is taking us. Obviously the MoHSS needed an evidence-based workforce assessment.

Shortly thereafter I received a letter from the Permanent Secretary (PS) asking IntraHealth Namibia through USAID to conduct a workforce assessment using the WHO tool called Workload Indicators of Staffing Need (WISN) in Kavango Region (one of the 13 regions of the country). Although I had never personally used the WISN tool to estimate the number of health workers needed, I had previously done some time-motion studies and understood what it was supposed to do. In just a couple of weeks we had collected and analyzed the data for doctors, nurses, pharmacists, and pharmacy assistants for all health facilities in the region and presented the results at the regional and national level. I made a recommendation to do a similar assessment for all regions so that the MoHSS would have concrete evidence for the restructuring process and to know how many health workers were needed to pick up the HIV/AIDS-related work.

Given the positive results at a regional level, the Deputy PS requested our support for a national WISN assessment at all public and faith-based health facilities in the country (345) for all doctors, nurses, pharmacists, and pharmacy assistants. Conducting this type of national assessment required a team of human resource experts, a WISN consultant to assist with the assessment, as well as clinical and information system experts. After several months I was able to present the results to the Minister of Health, PS, Deputy PS, and all national and regional directors within the health sector. The Ministry of Finance—upon seeing the results—said to the Director of Human Resources Development, "With these kinds of data I can see why you need additional staff." These findings were recently presented at the Global Health Workforce Alliance Meeting in Recife, Brazil, and published in the *Human Resources for Health Journal*.

SHARING STORIES

Road Trip

I have described my work as it unfolded over the past 30+ years to create a rich career. I want to now share a few stories that get at the heart of what I do.

One of my first trips after completing my PhD was to Haiti, where I conducted an evaluation of a family planning training that had been implemented by FHI a few months earlier. This involved developing a sub-agreement with a research firm in Haiti to assist in data collection, data input, analysis, and report writing. When we were ready to collect data I went along with the team of two nurses and two sociologists. I was surprised when the two nurses got into the car complaining about it being a sedan instead of a 4 × 4. They proceeded to put on back and neck braces as I looked at them strangely. I'll never forget their comment, "*Pamela tu verras*" (Pamela you will see). Shortly thereafter we headed for what looked like a mountain and I realized that we were indeed going to cross that mountain without any real roads. We were tossed about from side to side and within a short time had our first flat tire. Over the course of the week we had about six flats. We also had to cross a river in the car, sleep on the floor of a room full of mosquitoes as there were no hotels, and eat whatever food could be found since there were no restaurants. On one of our treks we found a bus that had overturned. Passengers were sitting along the side of the road. Naïvely, I took a picture and quickly had people yelling at me because (I was told) it was perceived that "the picture could see into their souls." After that I asked for permission before snapping pictures of interesting sights. There were a host of experiences in Haiti concerning voodoo and evil spirits. On one occasion, as we were collecting data, I tried out some of my Creole with the children in the village. Our driver said, "Do not ever turn your back away from these children so their parents cannot see you, if these children fall sick they will think you cast an evil spirit on them and they will come and get you."

Always a Solution

On another trip to Haiti I learned that I needed to be solution focused when the anticipated advance site preparation did not happen as expected. In this particular study, our local consultant was supposed to have contacted our sample health facilities to let them know the dates that we were coming to collect data and conduct focus group interviews with women who had had a tubal ligation in the previous 6 months. Our local consultant insisted that the groundwork had occurred. When we arrived at our first health facility to conduct the interviews, I learned that no one there had been informed that we were coming. Since this was the first time I had this experience, I immediately thought, "Oh my goodness we have wasted all of this money and time to come to Haiti with a team of data collectors and we can't do anything."

I talked to the nurse midwife in charge of the health facility, and upon hearing my concerns she said, "No problem, we will just announce it on the radio tonight and the women will come in tomorrow." I was quite the skeptic and thought that there was no way that the women who had a tubal ligation at this health center are going to happen to listen to the radio tonight and come in for the interviews tomorrow. I expected that either no one would show up or women who did not have the procedure would show up.

The next morning I woke up to a queue of women lined up outside of the health facility. I remained skeptical about who these women were. Fortunately, my skepticism proved to be unfounded as I pulled the medical records of the focus group participants and found that each woman had had a tubal ligation performed in the past 6 months at that particular health center.

When we went out to the second site, we had a similar finding. None of the staff on the ground were informed. At this particular site, the staff suggested that we send the driver with a loudspeaker to the village and make an announcement about what we needed. I totally doubted that this solution could work, but we had nothing to lose. Would you believe that I was wrong again? After a short period of time the driver came back with three car loads of women who apparently met the criteria. Again, we checked all of the medical records at the health center and found that these women indeed had had the procedure done in the last 6 months.

After that I had numerous experiences where I learned to rely on local expertise for innovative solutions when it appeared that all would fail. I cannot anticipate the issue or the solution, but I have learned to trust that a positive, credible outcome is achievable.

A Difficult Decision

I was confronted once with an incident in Haiti that challenged my research ethics. I was conducting another study on the quality of care regarding tubal ligation services. Being a good researcher I looked at the primary data on the individuals we were going to interview. I happened to notice that there were a lot of missing data about the date of the last menstrual cycle before the tubal ligation. I asked the data collectors to add a question about last menstrual cycle in their focus group discussions with women. Much to my surprise, several of the women talked about delivering a baby after they had their tubal ligation. They assumed that the method failed. In the following focus group discussions I continued to hear similar stories about a presumed method failure.

Our last site visit included direct observation at a small clinic being set up to conduct tubal ligations for a day. As we pulled up to the site there was a queue of women lined up outside. The clinic consisted of only one or two small rooms, no electricity, and no water. It was quite basic, to put it mildly. I was beginning to understand creole quite well. There were two nurses asking/telling the women that they didn't want to have more children, right??? The women usually nodded their head in agreement as they put ink on their thumb to make an imprint on the form indicating their agreement. They did not know how to sign their names. The nurses didn't ask any questions about the women's last menstrual cycle, explain about what to expect from the procedure, or attempt to find out what questions the women might have. The thumb print documented their informed consent. I was pretty sure that the presumed "method failure" was because many women were already pregnant when they came to the clinic to get the tubal ligation. So remembering everything I could about human subjects and research ethics, I decided to break my "observation" and ask the doctor about what I was seeing. I asked him a question like, "How do you know that these women are not pregnant when you perform the procedure?" I will never forget the shocked look on his face when he looked at the forms with missing dates of last menstrual cycle. He had only looked at the thumb print assuming that the nurses were only referring appropriate patients. The doctor then insisted that the nurses ask ALL the questions.

So now what do I do with the information that the procedures were being performed, most likely, on women who were already pregnant? After talking it over with a Haitian colleague, I decided that I needed to share my findings with the Haitian Minister of Health. It was a difficult decision because I knew that the services would be stopped once the Minister of Health heard about these findings. On the other hand, I could not let them continue to conduct tubal ligations on women who were already pregnant. I might add that the procedure does not hurt the unborn infant. My concern was the ethics surrounding selection criterion for clients receiving the medical procedure. To this day, I believe I made the correct decision.

Are We Dealing With the Right Issues?

On several occasions I've had the chance to travel to regions in Uganda and Southern Sudan that had experienced years of civil war. My purpose was to help improve human resources for health, but I realized we were really dealing with the residual hurt of the community from the effects of war. I would look at the blank, emotionless faces of many health workers and wonder about the trauma they were suffering.

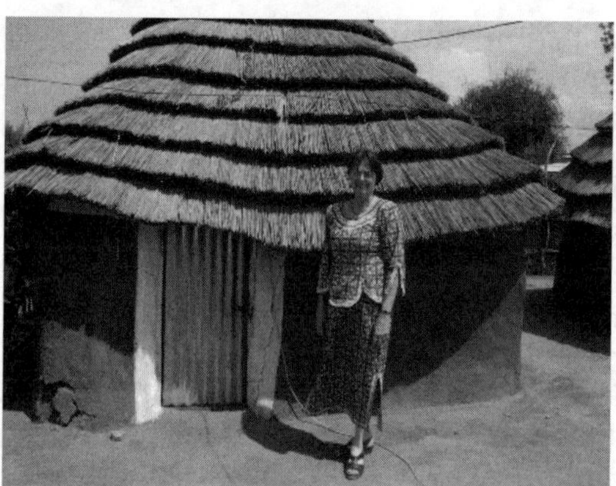

Figure 20.1 One of the Southern Sudan State Health Minister's guest houses where I spent the night. Photo by author.

One day I traveled with the Chief Nurse, Janet Michels, from Southern Sudan. The peace accord had been recently signed. We drove to one of the poorest areas. There were no real roads. We had to travel with an armed guard, and there was roadside evidence of blown up army trucks and tanks. We stopped to take a short break and noticed a handful of children playing nearby. As we got closer to them we realized they were climbing on a bomb that had not exploded. No one seemed to pay any attention to the fact that this was a real bomb. An aide worker from Kenya was also there and equally alarmed. We tried to get the authorities to remove the bomb and stop the children from playing in that area.

That night, Janet Michels and I shared one of the health minister's "huts" (pictured above) that he had recently constructed for guests visiting his state. Janet and I stayed up talking about what Sudan used to be like before the war. She said that when she was a young girl (before the war) Sudan was a wonderful and safe place to live. You could walk anywhere and knock on any door and people would take you in, offer you a meal, and allow you to stay if you needed a place to rest. There were no issues of insecurity. At that time women did not drink alcohol. She recalled a conversation with a friend recently where they discussed how things have changed after years of war. Women were now drinking and had a high rate of alcohol abuse. Janet's friend said, "But what didn't we see and experience during the war—how many of us weren't raped and beaten and saw people killed in front of our eyes?"

That conversation is still very real to me. I asked myself, "How can we hope to make real improvement when we are not dealing with the psychological scars of war?" People in these communities continue to face violence, rape, insecurity, and substance abuse as a secondary effect of the wars they experienced. How can they maximize their potential under these circumstances? The number of social workers and mental health professionals in most African countries is so limited that they rarely get out of the main offices in their capital cities. Schools of nursing and other health professions schools do not provide training regarding psychosocial support or good communication techniques. We need to keep asking ourselves, are we really dealing with issues that will make a difference?

MAKING A DIFFERENCE

Working With International Colleagues

Many of us consider global health work because we want to make a difference. We believe that health officials in the host country want our help, and we have the answers. Yet we do not realize that many international donors are knocking at the very same doors that we are and offering various types of international assistance. Some are luring officials with offers of travel and per diems to interesting countries around the world. Why should someone listen to me? Who can I trust? I obviously never took a class to teach me how to do this kind of work. Yet, I somehow subliminally figured out how to work with colleagues in many ministries of health.

First of all, it is all about relationships, trust, and networks. I remember when IntraHealth International did not have an office in Uganda. We wanted to see if USAID and the Ministry of Health were interested in technical assistance from us in human resources for health through the Capacity Project. We initially had to gather intelligence about the country, issues, what organizations were there and what were they doing, and hire a consultant that knew people in the MoH to get appointments for us. Without a consultant we could not have gotten in some of the doors. I also knew the Registrar at the Nursing Council from previous ECSA meetings and could get a meeting with her. So little by little we started to develop a web of relationships. These same busy people are inundated by groups of other donor agencies. Trust is critical. Staying in touch via e-mail rarely works. Face-to-face interactions over time are usually the most effective but often hard to do because of distance. Having local staff/consultants on the ground that you stay in touch with and who can follow up for you is very important.

I learned early on that not everyone in positions of power really want to make a difference in their country. Some are simply looking for personal gain in their interaction with you. I try to figure out who are the few people genuinely interested in making improvements. I focus on them. I have had several difficult experiences where I was told publically at a meeting, "Pamela you do not facilitate us the way other partners do," meaning I don't give them "top-ups" (bribes). I refuse to give in to pressure to do so, but realize my actions may make it difficult or impossible for me to work in a particular country. Do not compromise on your ethics. If someone is only interested in his or her own personal gain, this person is not going to follow up after you leave. The problem is that small "top-ups" are so prevalent in some places that people do not see it as a bribe. It is just a way of doing business.

Looking back, I cannot remember a country in which I have worked where there are not organizations and government health officials that really want to make improvements. They appreciate honest, trustworthy experts who can help them achieve their goals for their country. Development work involves listening to the needs and potential solutions identified by internal stakeholders and then in supporting them to become successful. Do not think that because of your degrees and experience that you are going to come in and have all the answers. They may take your money, but the chance that it will lead to sustainable development it unlikely. I am always thrilled when a final report comes out with the names of the Ministry of Health officials listed and my name is listed somewhere in the back. This shows that they have taken ownership of the results.

I have found it very helpful when collaborating with nurses and other health professionals to share that I am a nurse during initial introductions. An early economic study that I did in Kenya about ability and willingness to pay for family planning services involved interviews with nurses and clients. I can remember arriving at one of the health facilities and introducing myself to the hospital manager, saying I am also a nurse. "Let me show you my unit" was the response as the manager proceeded to show me around the hospital and introduced me to all the nurses we needed to work with. I usually reserve the "I am Dr. Pamela McQuide" for when I first meet with high-level officials at the Ministry of Health and they need to know that I have a certain level of qualification that gets me in the door. But these occasions are fairly infrequent. Besides, my business card lists all those details.

Lessons Learned

After all these years of working in global health I have learned a few lessons.

- *If I cannot find a way to make a difference and if there is no country ownership, I won't waste my time. I refuse to compromise my ethics.*
- *Too many Americans come in and think that we have all of the answers and try to tell people what they have to do. They don't realize that the colleagues with which we are working actually have the answers.*
- *It is most gratifying to combine local expertise with my experience (from nursing, management, research, and policy) and come up with an answer that combines all these lessons learned.*
- *Frequently in the midst of trying to implement a study or intervention it appears that things will not work. I have learned to relax and realize that a solution will be found that is credible, but it is never one that could have been anticipated.*
- *Some of the adverse issues we cope with are due to the mistakes of previous donors.*
- *More nurses with advanced degrees should do global health. We understand health care delivery and we know how to work as a team player.*
- *My training did not prepare me for doing global health research or international development kind of work.*
- *One needs to consistently be on the look-out for potential fraud and corruption. We need to set up strict accountability systems to prevent those who want to do the right thing from making poor choices.*
- *Understanding the political context and political relationships is essential to knowing who really has the power to do what.*

Preparation for Global Health Nursing

I think that nurses are uniquely qualified to do global health. We understand health settings and we work well in teams. When I worked at FHI my colleagues often expressed envy of my nursing background because I knew how to work with health workers and I understood what health care services should look like.

However, I do not think that many schools of nursing prepare students for a career path in global health. We do a great job of ensuring that the clinical practice and research skills of our graduates meet high standards, but we do little to teach potential international development workers how to work in diverse settings. Key areas of preparations should include how to identify the groups in the country who can support research activities; how to conduct trainings with transfer of learning methods; how to train and supervise teams of data collectors and data entrants; how to build capacity of local partners so their skills are increased, thereby improving the possibility for sustainability; how to identify and ensure country ownership of strategies; how to develop memorandums of understanding between different stakeholder groups; how to set up systems to pay for trainings and research studies; and to recognize fraudulent bids and claim the list goes on and on.

I would encourage anyone who wants to do international health work to apply for an internship. I have had interns work with me on several occasions and they are usually a win-win. When I taught a master's level class to nurses interested in international health at Emory University, each student had to develop an international project with a mentor where they got to actually participate in a research or training type of project. Two of the students traveled to Kenya with me to collect data for an HIV study. They were paired with master's students at a Kenyan university to help implement the study. This gave the master's students hands-on experience and I had support to conduct the study.

Hope for the Future

My hope is that nurses everywhere will recognize the valuable contributions they make to improve the health of their communities. I want them to be proud of being nurses and to see nursing as an important career choice. This may be even more important in developing countries than it is in the United States, where the work of nurses is often not recognized and there are few leaders in key government positions with a nursing background. I want nurses to see that they too can get a doctorate and make important contributions to the health systems of their countries.

It has been a privilege to do the work that I do; to collaborate with amazing partners in challenging settings. It's been a rewarding career choice and I feel blessed.

21

Nous Sommes Ensemble

We Are Together

RUTH-ANNE McLENDON

Editor's Note: We close the collection with Ruth-Anne McLendon's guidance regarding preparation for global health nursing. Ruth-Anne draws on the literature and heart-warming personal stories to illustrate practical skills-building strategies. Her lessons learned will resonate with readers as we reflect on discussions of previous writers that support and illustrate her points. This chapter evolved from Ruth-Anne's undergraduate honors thesis.

I walked home from the hospital after the first day, through the dusty hot town, past the ladies selling peanuts and the young men riding around on their motorcycles. I walked past the potholes in the dirt road and women chatting over their mats covered in mangos. I walked into the cool interior of my host-family's house and tears started to flow. I felt incompetent, useless, and shy.

My day had begun as one might expect. I had arrived in Thies, Senegal, a few days earlier, prepared to work at a local private hospital for the summer. This day, I climbed from under my mosquito net-draped bed and shuffled over the tile floor. I picked out a skirt and shirt and then ate my egg and baguette breakfast, prepared by my gracious host mother.

At the hospital, I sat on the bed in the nurse's station, halfway watching the television and partly trying to make conversation while not understanding most of what was being said. I asked awkward and strange American questions:

"How many children do you have?" (Later, I discovered this is akin to calling down curses on someone.)

"How do you like being a nurse?"

"How many languages do you speak?" (The answer would often be four or five, to my amazement.)

"Why did you want to work here?" (Many people could not find work and so were doing unpaid internships in hopes of improving their chances of employment.)

I tried to be useful. It complicates instructions when you don't know what people are telling you to do; you wouldn't know how or where to do it even if you did understand, and you don't know why the patients are being treated the way they are. I was in culture shock, disoriented and overwhelmed by the newness around me and discouraged by the language barrier.

My interests in global health and cross-cultural nursing began early. As the daughter of missionaries, I spent my early years growing up in Belgium and Niger, West Africa. I was exposed to different cultures and different ways of doing things. I grew up seeing the differences between us and the neighbors living in stick and mud houses. The food, the language, and even the way people greeted each other were different.

Now I was returning to West Africa as a nursing student and the transition was challenging. I flew into Dakar, Senegal, alone, with nothing but the names of several contacts, a suitcase, and a laptop. The opportunity to volunteer at the hospital had come about in a roundabout way. After deciding to participate in a global health course offered by my school of nursing, I met a missionary nurse who had worked at the hospital in Thies. She connected me with the Senegalese organization that runs the hospital. They accepted my application, and several months later I found myself in Dakar and on my way to Thies.

There are things I wish I had known before I arrived, and ways the transition could have been easier. Cross-cultural nursing and cross-cultural living are complex, multilayered, exhausting, and fundamental to global health.

Perhaps you are thinking about traveling to a different country, or working with people from a different background or language. This chapter is intended to help you peel back some of those layers, and answer questions such as, what can cross-cultural nursing look like? How do we break down barriers to best care for patients? How do we prepare ourselves to work in a cross-cultural health care setting? We can start by examining ourselves, then examining cultural differences and similarities. We can learn how to communicate, forge new relationships, and work together toward better health care for our patients.

REFLECT: CHECKING ASSUMPTIONS

> "You can't help but learn your biases when you are so immersed in another culture. And you learn a lot about what you take for granted. For example, you take for granted that people understand you in certain ways and of course, they don't, so you have to try to be resourceful and think about how you could get them to understand."
>
> Quote from a Western expatriate nurse educator working in East Asia (Melby, Dodgson & Tarrant, 2008, p. 180).

Spending time in a different culture has a way of challenging the way you view your own cultural background and the traditions of the people you are surrounded by. Sharing similar backgrounds can aid in making connections because people unconsciously operate with "shared assumptions and expectations" (Hearnden, 2008). Values differ between cultures and between individuals, and those differences can cause misunderstandings. The key word here is "assumptions." It is easy to make assumptions about people based on their background or culture, and it is equally easy to assume that someone's behavior means the same thing to them as it means to you. Culture impacts people's priorities and assumptions regarding health care.

The census of the small, private hospital where I found myself, despite being in the second-largest city in Senegal, was very low. Rising costs and changes in staff had contributed to a decline in patient admissions. The result was a lot of sitting around in the hospital when the patients stopped trickling in.

I was appalled at first. I felt a bit cheated, as if my student experience was going to be wasted. I wanted to get my hands dirty. I wanted to be of use. I wanted to help the poor people of Senegal. I wanted to be a hero.

I was frustrated with sitting around most afternoons and doing "nothing"—only chatting with the other Senegalese interns and watching overly dramatic soap operas badly dubbed into French.

I finally marched down to the hospital receptionist, a lovely lady named Constance. "I came here to work, not to sit around. I want to be useful." I said, in broken, emphatic French. Being one of the sweetest ladies I have ever met, she smiled and assured me she would find work for me to do. After that, nearly every time I saw her she asked if I had work to do. As time passed, I realized there was not much work for anyone except the physicians. I had arrogantly demanded work because "that is what I came to do," without recognizing my assumption that of course I would be useful.

Subconsciously, I assumed that I could do something that the Senegalese people working there could not do. Later, I realized that the way I handled the situation—while politely received—was very direct, confrontational, and smelled strongly of a Western, fast-paced, get-it-done-and-don't-waste-time attitude. My assumptions were based on my background and values that define me by my work. I now understand that there was an underlying belief that what I accomplished was more important than the people with whom I accomplished it.

Once I came to that realization, I stopped trying to define myself by the number of injections I administered or the number of wound dressings I changed. I was able to savor time spent with the other interns and nurses. I was then able to gain more insight into their view of the world.

While this is just one example of how my culture affected my attitude, there are many others that you may encounter while working with a group of people who are different from you. To successfully work with those groups, it is helpful to carefully consider what is meant by the term "cultural competence." Dr. Josepha Campinha-Bacote, a nursing theorist, developed a 5-step model of cultural competence in health care services delivery. The model includes cultural awareness, cultural skill, cultural knowledge, cultural encounters, and cultural desire (Dayer-Berenson, 2011, p. 30). Campinha-Bacote's model of cultural competence helps respond to questions such as, how do you work with clients and health care workers from other cultures in a way that is sensitive and maximizes patient benefit?

I will refer to the concept of "culture" throughout this chapter, even though it is an imperfect term that covers traditions, lifestyles, and values espoused by different groups of people. While there are many definitions of culture, most definitions include two components: shared and learned knowledge and values, and a community in which they operate (Hearnden, 2008, p. 51). Culture is something that is "learned and passed on within a group" (Jirwe, Gerrish & Emami, 2010, p. 442). While culture is stereotypically linked with an ethnic identity or citizenship, it is also used to describe aspects of smaller subgroups of people, for example, the homeless community (Jirwe et al., 2010, p. 442).

Values, on the other hand, represent "a way of life and give direction to life," and they are developed through interacting with others (Parfitt, 1994).

Cultural awareness, the first component of Campinha-Bacote's model, addresses self-examination: What are my biases and traditions? How do they affect the way that I look at people of other cultures, traditions, and value systems? How does it impact the health care services that are delivered?

Enhancing cultural awareness requires confronting our beliefs and taking the time to become aware of the culture and values we have internalized. Cultural awareness is a tool that can be used to better relate to people of different backgrounds, whether or not they are of the same ethnicity. Cultural awareness is about examining the significance of our assumptions and biases.

Many values are subconscious and are accepted without question. For instance, I learned that I had internalized a value that mandates task—completion in order to achieve success—one that says "time is money." In order to be productive, one must do something tangible (such as giving an injection). With this school of thought, sitting and chatting is not productive and therefore a waste of time.

Hearnden, in an article about cross-cultural communication, argues that people communicate with a certain set of assumptions and expectations. Misunderstanding between the nurse and clients increases when those expectations and values do not match (Hearnden, 2008, p. 51). Differences in customs and traditions can create misunderstandings about the deeper feelings of the individuals involved.

It is easy to make judgments of people different than yourself based on customs, appearance, and presuppositions. A 2010 study polled the experiences of Filipino and Ghanaian nurses working in the United Kingdom. Topics discussed included making assumptions about patients' relatives based on their actions.

"I wondered—what sort of culture is this? What kind of cruelty is this? They believe that even though their relative is in the hospital, they can check on them over the phone without coming to the hospital."

"I have found that [British] people are not really attached the way we are to our relatives" (Okougha & Tilki 2010).

The article goes on to discuss the responses of nurses to cross-cultural experiences with death, dying, demonstrating respect, and being polite. There was a lot of room for misunderstanding in these situations, and the participants' views were usually based on their own experiences and values (Okougha & Tilki, 2010).

Shortly after I arrived in Senegal, a good friend of my host mother lost someone close to her. My host mother, along with several of her friends, prepared to visit Julie to comfort her. They invited me to join them. I was taken aback. I did not know Julie and I did not feel comfortable going, so I decided against it. Later I realized how important "being with" was in the culture, a principle component of Kristen Swanson's theory of caring (Swanson, 1998). If I could do it over, I would go and be present to show caring to her, even though my culture does not deal with death in that way. My cultural frame of reference was different than the one in operation at that moment, so the result was a potential social faux pas and loss of trust. Fortunately, my host mother and the other women were very understanding of my feelings and it did not appear to cause a problem. However, if they had assumed I was not present because I did not care about Julie or her grief, then it could have created major barriers in our relationship.

As noted above, the concept of cultural awareness is designed to encourage self-awareness and contemplation of personal values and culture, which will lead to open-minded interactions with people of different backgrounds. But how do we foster cultural awareness?

The researchers who talked with the Filipino and Ghanaian nurses recommended that coworkers and supervisors give gentle reminders of socially acceptable behavior (Okougha & Tilki, 2010). Finding an ally who can act as a cultural broker helps pick up on the cues. Cultural brokers are people who are very familiar with customs and traditions in more than one setting. They often know what to do and what not to do and can help with understanding the reasoning behind why things are done a certain way (Burger, 2011).

The Westerners as all-knowing saviors belief can be tempting, especially when considering cross-cultural health care (Parfitt, 1994). Because a major motivation can be altruism, it is possible to go inspired to fix, to do, to make better. While this is not necessarily bad in and of itself, cultural and self-awareness are important in achieving balanced decision-making and "helping." Working closely with and for local communities and health services instead of "fixing" them are key.

At the root of cultural awareness is humility. As an outsider and a novice nurse, I was not prepared to know the best way to care for my Senegalese patients. I had to learn how to enter with an attitude of openness to learning and self-reflection. A fellow nursing student who enrolled in the same global health course that facilitated my trip to Senegal wrote, "I would tell any student to just go with an open mind and open heart. Take in all that you see, smell, hear, taste and touch. Do not judge since you do not know."[1]

EXPLORE: STUDYING CULTURE

> "I think that people traveling abroad should learn about the history of the country as much as possible before going. Because once I understood the history, the health care setting, the culture of the people, and lack of resources made so much more sense . . ."
>
> UNC Chapel Hill nursing student, after participating in the global health experience.

Differences in expectations, customs, and lifestyle influence how smoothly one adjusts to another culture and customs. Many authors have discussed an experience called "culture shock," defined as "a series of common cognitive and emotional reactions to transcultural immersion" (Melby et al., 2008, p. 181). Differences in customs, traditions, relationships, language, and the way things are done can be overwhelming and confusing, necessitating relearning many life skills, and practicing coping skills.

My first week in Senegal was physically and mentally exhausting. The heat affected my energy level. I was constantly aware of my words and actions and afraid of giving offense. I was always aware of my skin color. I could not understand people very well and had trouble communicating. I blundered through greetings. I was very unsure of myself when communicating with men, because I did not want to offend Muslim traditions. If I had to describe the first few weeks with one word, I would say "uncomfortable." Sleeping under a mosquito net, ignoring the catcalls of men in the street, wearing long skirts, and eating bone-in fish were new to me. Everything had to be relearned. Most of the discomfort came from not knowing and feeling unsure.

Becoming familiar with what to do and what not to do lessens the "not-knowing" aspect of culture shock. That being said, I found that there were values and customs that I did not know about, and had I known about them earlier my path would have been much smoother—issues like asking for gifts, for example.

The Senegalese people seem to have very different attitudes toward possessions than Westerners do, or at least than I do. Interactions surrounding them caused me to learn more about my own perspective and attitudes. Early in my time at the hospital I made friends with a nurse who was completing a 3-month internship. Yacine and I often worked together as we rotated through the different areas of the hospital. The first time she asked me for my scrubs I was caught off guard. I was wearing blue scrubs that had cost about $10 at Walmart, but they looked very new compared to the scrubs the staff wore.

"Ruth, you are going to give me that shirt when you leave, right?"

The shirt was new, not bleach-stained, and had pants with it, therefore the scrubs looked really nice. I laughed it off. She continued to ask me for the scrubs, sometimes jokingly, sometimes seriously.

After I returned to the United States, she sent a message asking for money to resolve a legal issue. Her request for both the scrubs and later for money was disconcerting. My impression of a person who asks for such things is that he or she is needy, demanding, lazy, or rude. Then I began to think. Asking for gifts is a phenomenon that does not necessarily mean the same thing to people with different backgrounds. Complicating that thought was the fact that, compared to her, I do have more resources.

I asked for advice. I talked with my host mother and with my father who has experience living in West Africa. They offered ideas about the basis for her requests and the best way to proceed. I ended up giving all my scrubs to one of the staff nurses at the hospital and asked her to distribute them to the other nurses. I did not send my friend money after I returned home.

Clearly, attitudes and behaviors involving gifts and a host of other issues are complicated. While I had had some inkling of this fact beforehand, I was not prepared to deal with it without help. Therefore, this portion of the chapter is designed to help you ask for help.

What do you need to know? What do you need to ask about? We take a lot for granted—how to greet someone, how to pay someone, how to ask questions, how to answer questions. People with different backgrounds have different assumptions about what to expect. This especially applies to health care workers because of differences in how care is provided and expectations surrounding that care.

Where do you start? When providing health care, it is important to have an understanding about a patient's background. Campinha-Bacote describes this as "cultural knowledge"—one component of cultural competency. Enhancing cultural knowledge entails gathering sound information that will help provide care when working cross-culturally (Dayer-Berenson, 2011). A cultural broker can help you do that.

While I lived in Senegal, I had several cultural brokers. An American couple taught me it was generally appropriate to shake hands to greet others. However, they cautioned that I should wait for men to extend their hands in greeting first, in case they were conservative Muslims and prohibited from touching women. My host mother, a very gracious Zambian lady, taught me a lot as well. While neither the couple nor my host mother was Senegalese, they had a great deal of experience with Senegalese customs, and being outsiders, had had to learn those things for themselves. In addition, I had friends who worked at the hospital—other interns and nurses—who provided insight into the Senegalese way of doing things.

Having cultural brokers, especially ones who understand differences between Senegalese and Western life, was very helpful. They were able to help me anticipate what to expect and what to prepare myself for. Cultural brokers can help with preparation for your time in another culture or country, process your experiences once you get there, and help debrief when you return home.

Analyzing Culture

How do you go about learning what you need to know? Giger and Davidhizar's transcultural assessment model identifies six different cultural phenomena that they argue shape health care and provide a framework for assessing and learning about culture. According to them, these six factors provide necessary information for providing "culturally discordant" care (Dayer-Berenson, 2011, p. 21). These six factors are communication, space, social organization, time, environmental control, and biologic variations.

Communication, discussed more fully later in this chapter, is defined broadly as human interaction—speech and nonverbal communication—which is shaped by culture (Dayer-Berenson, 2011, p. 23). Space refers to the unspoken rules surrounding personal space and the polite distance between people during interactions. Time orientation reflects interpersonal communication regarding how time is viewed. There is a proverb that I heard while in Senegal, "Westerners have watches, but Africans have time." Some cultures value appointment-oriented time while others focus on people and events, not clocks. Environmental control describes how people view and control events. Beliefs about control over health status effect patient attitudes toward self-care. The last category, biological variation, considers genetic differences between groups and formulates the best practices for responding to those differences (Dayer-Berenson, 2011, pp. 23–26).

I have discussed Giger and Davidhizar's model because I think it can help focus the search for cultural knowledge and can provide structure for questions to discuss with your cultural broker. Suspending judgment and asking good questions will smooth the path of learning.

Differences in Health Care Practices

As many of the contributors to this book have pointed out, there are many differences in how health care is provided around the world. Clinician roles, staff interactions, resource allocation, sanitation, pain management, and many other factors influence care. Cultural brokers helped me to understand that the differences I observed in Senegal are closely interconnected and affect each other as well as the health care system as a whole.

Nursing Roles

The nurses that I worked with at the hospital had a very different view of their role as nurses than I did. There appeared to be more focus on tasks such as medication administration and dressing changes, and less emphasis on patient assessment. In the United States, nurses' aides and nurses assist patients with personal care. In Senegal, family members stay with patients at all times to help with feeding, bathing, and toileting.

Resource Allocation

Because of the lower socioeconomic status of patients and the financial difficulties of the hospital, resources were not readily available. Once, when I asked for hand sanitizer, the nurse gave me a small bottle but told me to use it sparingly, as it was expensive.

In another instance, I assisted with the catheterization of a postoperative patient. She was overweight and it was difficult to catheterize her. The nurses started with one catheter and used a clean, not sterile technique. Several nurses tried, using the same catheter. Finally, on the third or fourth attempt the nurse manager was successful—using the same catheter.

These anecdotes illustrate the balance between resources and hygiene. While many of the nurses had a concept of clean and sterile technique, decisions were not made solely on evidence-based practice. Practical issues were important, for instance, how will the patient pay for this? Can the patient afford another catheter? How can we save money? Often the availability of resources swayed the decision. I saw trays with blood products and dressings from infected wounds being wiped down with alcohol and used for subsequent patients. I felt uncomfortable at times, because it seemed that by trying to protect the patient from infection I was perceived as being wasteful. I realize the nurses' actions were not intended to harm the patient. They were just trying to make the care affordable for the patient and to keep the hospital afloat, financially. Navigating these constraints requires adaptability and innovation—maintaining hygienic practices while improving resource conservation.

Nursing students who participated in the global health course in other areas of the world made similar observations. When asked, a common theme was resource allocation. Their comments reflected frugality and learning to being resourceful.

"The Project reused everything. They washed face masks and sheets for examining tables. The nurse in the clinic used the same thermometer for everyone without sterilizing in between."

"I was surprised that the foundations of health care practices were very similar to practices in the United States. However, the resources were extremely limited in the clinic, and I was surprised how the health care workers adapted."

"I . . . learned how to use the resources that I had to provide care. For example, we had to save linens whenever possible. So sometimes we used extra chux pads to prevent stains in the sheets."

Resources are precious—something that health workers in U.S. hospitals may not be as conscious of. Working in areas with low resources requires adaptation and ingenuity.

Traditional Medicine

One morning I worked in the Salle de Pansements, which was the room where we performed outpatient dressing changes. We had a string of patients that morning, from lacerations to burns. Mid-morning, an older woman in a long dress and wrapped in a veil walked in. When she sat down in the chair, we unwrapped her head dressing and found a series of masses growing on her head and face. The largest one was on her cheek, firm to palpation and about the size of a small orange. She needed a dressing change because the mass had an open, scabbed-over wound. Using our hand-folded and sterilized gauze pads, I started cleaning the wound. As I gently loosened the scabs and washed the wound, I began to pull out hair. It was not short facial hairs or the soft curly hair that grew on her head. The strands were about a foot long, and appeared to be horse hair. We were not the first healers she had gone to for help.

In my experience, living in Niger as a young child, the local hospital was the place where people went to die. After exhausting all other options, sacrificing to demons, and seeking healing in other places, they would come to the hospital and their prophecy of death would often be self-fulfilling because they were so late in seeking care. Traditional medicine may be more trusted. It is also often tied with religion and spirituality. It is important, therefore, to explore what other venues of healing your patients are using.

Religion and Spirituality

In Senegal, 95% of the population is conservative Muslim. During my time there, Ramadan, the month of fasting, began. During Ramadan, people fast from dawn until dusk, breaking the fast in the evening. Women get up in the middle of the night to cook a meal before dawn, and then everyone except young children, pregnant women, and the sick go without food during the daylight hours. This is one example of a religious tradition that affects health care—strict Muslims will not even drink water during the day. Nutritional issues due to fasting and fatigue affect health status and are important considerations when working with patients.

These are just a few examples of how culture can affect health care; both the way it is administered and the way it is viewed. A cultural broker can help you be better prepared for what to expect and how to respond. Cultural brokers can also help you learn how to better communicate with your patients and coworkers.

This brings us to the last category in cultural competence and adaptation. As discussed above, one of Giger and Davidhizar's cultural phenomena is communication. It is essential to connecting with patients and caring for them.

TALK: COMMUNICATING AND CONNECTING

My first experience with cross-cultural communication was in Belgium. I was 2 years old, newly enrolled in preschool, surrounded by French-speakers. I remember Madame Claire; a flash of blond hair, red lipstick, and a loud voice. I did not speak or understand French, and while she knew that, her method of ensuring that I understood was to speak louder. I spent my first preschool days being yelled at in a language that I did not understand. The language barrier caused me to believe she was angry with me, which prevented me from participating in class and activities. Her method of handling the language barrier alienated me and prevented a productive relationship from developing for a long time.

Flash-forward to my time in Senegal where I encountered communication issues from the start. My 4 years of French in high school with another four semesters slogging through French in college—an experience that I was sure had made me practically fluent—fell disappointingly flat. The combination of being less competent with the language than expected plus a new accent caused a lot of headaches for me and the people I attempted to speak with. To top it off, I had not anticipated that the majority of patients spoke only passable French.

In Senegal, there are two national languages—French and Wolof. Wolof is the universal trading and communication language. Most, if not all, Senegalese have a grasp of Wolof. French, on the other hand, is the language of the government, colonialism, and the educational system. I found that mainly individuals with higher levels of education spoke fluent French. Many of the patients I helped care for were not well educated and therefore did not speak much French.

I used the down time at the hospital to ask friends for words and phrases in Wolof. I wrote them in a notebook and practiced them whenever I had a chance. Still, it was not enough to actually have a conversation with a patient. I could say simple greetings and instructions ("How is your family?" "Please step onto the scale") but was frustrated in my efforts to really connect with patients. I could smile at them but I could not express myself fully.

I did not realize how vital verbal communication is until I suddenly could not communicate. Communication is important in any context where you are interacting with another human being, but it is vital for patient care. In any culture, you have to communicate with your patients to connect with them, to identify their needs, to assess their health history, to collaborate with them on treatment plans, to teach about treatments and care, and to do a host of other things (Jirwe et al., 2010). If you do not have the proper vocabulary, you cannot even ask the patient whether he or she needs more blankets or would like a glass of water.

Gestures

Body language—including gestures—contains a plethora of cues that can communicate very different things to people with different backgrounds. Before I arrived in Senegal, I learned that the left hand is considered the "dirty" hand. To use your left hand to eat, accept gifts, shake hands, or perform other actions was considered rude. I could give someone a beautiful gift, but if I offered it with my left hand it would be insulting to the recipient. If, on the other hand, I offered a gift to one of my American friends and extended it in my left hand, the gesture would mean nothing beyond the fact that I was giving them something. Cultural context interprets gestures. Gestures are tightly linked with conversation, and can reflect cultural values (Kita, 2009).

Emblem gestures (for example, giving a "thumbs up" motion) can mean different things in different cultures. Nodding your head may mean "yes" or agreement in Western culture. However, in Japanese culture it is a motion that signifies coordination and cooperation, but not necessarily agreement (Kita, 2009). Even spatial information can be communicated with different kinds of gestures based on how the language describes space. For example, the concept of "forward" and "back" for future and past are not common to all language groups and cultures (Kita, 2009).

Interpreting gestures and nuances shape communication and interpretation of communication. This is another area where it is important to consider your assumptions and observe closely—while something may seem obvious (to me it seems obvious that their nodding signifies agreement), simple gestures can communicate very different messages to different individuals.

When one considers communication, however, the first thought is usually in regard to language and the spoken word.

Language

Language can be a bridge or a barrier. Language differences can create a sense of separation. My teacher, Madame Claire, could not understand me and I could not understand her, so when she attempted to work with me toward a goal, it was ineffective. We were unable to connect and collaborate.

In health care, if the nurse and patient do not speak the same language, a barrier is created. This barrier results in lack of rapport (McCarthy, Cassidy, Graham & Tuohy, 2013) and understanding on both sides. Limited understanding can cause complications with assessments, teaching, treatment plans, and follow-up. If you cannot talk with your patient it is difficult to explore their health history (McCarthy et al., 2013). If you do not know his or her background, it is difficult to work toward treatment and healing.

Many health care facilities employ professional interpreters, though some rely on the patients' relatives. Engaging family members is not ideal because of issues involving confidentiality and sharing and withholding information (McCarthy et al., 2013). Sometimes nurses revert to creative communication such as gesturing, which doesn't work well either (McCarthy et al., 2013).

When I surveyed nursing students who had participated in the global health course, nearly all of them voiced regret at not being better prepared to speak the language of their patients. They consistently commented that language differences were difficult to navigate and complicated patient care.

I was involved with patient care at the hospital in Senegal, but with the language barrier it felt as if I were practicing with a handicap. Frustration was a frequent response to my inability to easily connect and collaborate. However, even though I could not speak more than a few phrases of Wolof, the language barrier softened when I made an effort to use what I was learning. Suddenly I was surrounded by "professors" who were eager to share their culture and background with me.

One afternoon, during my Wolof "lesson" with the nurses, another nurse came in and stood in the doorway for a few moments. "Toog" (sit down), I said, and motioned at the space next to me. She immediately burst out laughing and sat down. She was surprised to hear Wolof words come out of my mouth, but the fact that I uttered them created a connection between us.

By and large, the most common response I received (when it was not a blank stare caused by butchered pronunciation) was a wide smile, followed by, "Oh! You are learning Wolof!" By making an effort to learn Wolof, I was able to send a message that I found their language, and by extension them, valuable and worth learning about and caring for.

Making an effort to cross the communication barrier by examining nuances, gestures, and the meaning behind them, as well as by studying the language can do much to enhance connections with patients and coworkers. Those connections enable nurses to improve the level of care we provide and by extension improve patient health outcomes.

CONCLUSION

Throughout this chapter I have shared my experiences in Senegal in order to illustrate concepts regarding global health and cross-culture nursing. In doing so, I hope I have provided useful ideas for preparing to work among people whose life experience may be very different from your own. I began by discussing self-awareness and the importance of thinking through automatic assumptions. I mentioned the importance of viewing your patients not just as members of a cultural community but as individuals with a unique cultural make-up. And I talked about communication—crossing language and cultural barriers with patients and coworkers to promote understanding and cooperation. While this chapter provides pointers, immersion in another culture is a hugely illuminating experience that will teach you much more than a chapter in any book.

There is so much richness to be gained and given in cross-cultural nursing. Here is a summary of how you can use this chapter to prepare for your own unique experience:

1. Think about your attitudes, assumptions, biases, and values. How do they affect the health care that you provide?
2. Find cultural brokers. Perhaps you have a contact in the country where you are traveling. Find someone you can talk to, ask advice of, and process your experiences with. Try to find an insider as well as an experienced outsider.
3. Find out all you can about the country and culture you will be in contact with. Go through the different phenomenon of culture and talk with your cultural broker about them.
4. Do your homework: learn about the history of the region; read novels, histories, and biographies; listen to music; spend time learning the language even if you have access to interpreters. Every little bit helps!

Your global health experience will be made easier by embracing "curiosity, tolerance and appreciation for differences, acceptance of ambiguity, a sense of humor, low goal and task orientation, and knowing that failure is imminent" (Swanson, Goody, Frolova, Kuznetsova, Plavinski, & Nelson, 2001, p. 35). You will make mistakes, no matter how well you try to understand new traditions, but you will learn from them and grow as a person and as a nurse.

As I headed home after my first day at the hospital, my friend Jean attempted to describe the route to me in French. I was confused, my brain was tired, and my French comprehension was dwindling rapidly. I started walking in the wrong direction. Jean turned me around, making sure I understood how to get back to my host family.

"Don't worry," he said. "Nous sommes ensemble." While I did not appreciate what he meant at the time, I heard it again from several other Senegalese friends. They were telling me that we were in this together and that they would take care of me. They said it so matter-of-factly that I did not realize until later how serious they were about it. They went out of their way to take care of me. We grew closer as I learned to adapt to their hospitable culture and work in health care alongside them.

NOTES

1. The author conducted an anonymous survey of the other students who participated in the global health course described in the preface to this book.

REFERENCES

Burger, J. (2011). Diversity. A novel approach to increasing cultural awareness in novice nursing students. *Nurse Educator, 36*(3), 96–97.

Dayer-Berenson, L. (2011). *Cultural competencies for nurses.* Sudbury, MA: Jones and Bartlett Publishers, LLC.

Hearnden, M. (2008). Coping with differences in culture and communication in health care. *Nursing Standard, 23*(11), 49–58.

Jirwe, M., Gerrish, K., & Emami, A. (2010). Student nurses' experiences of communication in cross-cultural care encounters. *Scandinavian Journal of Caring Sciences, 24*(3), 436–444.

Kita, S. (2009). Cross-cultural variation of speech-accompanying gesture: A review. *Language & Cognitive Processes*, 24(2), 145–167.

McCarthy, J., Cassidy, I., Graham, M. M., & Tuohy, D. (2013). Conversations through barriers of language and interpretation. *British Journal of Nursing*, 22(6), 335–339.

Melby, C. S., Dodgson, J. E., & Tarrant, M. (2008). The experiences of western expatriate nursing educators teaching in eastern Asia. *Journal of Nursing Scholarship*, 40(2), 176–183.

Okougha, M., & Tilki, M. (2010). Experience of overseas nurses: The potential for misunderstanding. *British Journal of Nursing*, 19(2), 102–106.

Parfitt, B. (1994). Value orientations of expatriate nurses in the developing countries. *International Journal of Nursing Studies*, 31(3), 279–288.

Swanson, E., Goody, C. M., Frolova, E. V., Kuznetsova, O., Plavinski, S., & Nelson, G. (2001). An application of an effective interdisciplinary health-focused cross-cultural collaboration. *Journal of Professional Nursing*, 17(1), 33–39.

Swanson, K. (1998). Caring made visible. *Creative Nursing*, 4(4), 8.

Epilogue

Same Body, Different Rules

LAURA CALAMOS NASIR

They were absolutely incredulous. The nurses looked at me with absolute disbelief. Why would you have another person in the room?! So disrespectful of the patient's privacy!

I had taught history taking and physical examination for many years in the United States. This morning's session about pelvic examination went as expected. And yet, here I was in London, with a second set of nurses in the classroom telling me I was doing it all wrong.

Privacy and respect mean no extra people in the room. I couldn't argue with the logic. And yet having another nurse in the room was just what we did, what I taught, no matter the gender of the examiner. And so I came face to face with the bias of my first health care system. Like your first family, it had raised me to believe that there was a "right" way to do things. And so I was out in the world assuming everyone did it the same way—we are all humans after all. But of course, there are cultural differences even between us, English speakers. Health care systems are cultural phenomena like different tribes. Rules and policies develop differently; adapt to the variety of available resources. In the United Kingdom (according to the guidance notes laid out by the Royal College of Nursing), chaperones are to be "invited" to the pelvic exam when the appointment is made. They are there for the comfort of the woman and at her choice. In the United States, a second clinician accompanies the examiner, with no choice given to the female patient. We say it is for her safety, but we know it may protect us against potential "misunderstandings" (a.k.a., lawsuits); two different ways of understanding "protection."

And so the students taught the teacher. There is no "table" with "stirrups" for her feet—just a flat "couch." The speculum handle points up, not down (indeed the shape is designed to face this direction). And there is no stool to wheel up at eye level to her intimate areas—but a standing approach is made from the side and leaning over to examine. All these practical accommodations made sense for the type of (more affordable) equipment that was typically available in the National Health Service. The shock expressed by these experienced nurses—now advance practice students—at my every move woke me up, causing me to be self-conscious. Feeling like a novice nurse, I thought—Why do I do it this way? What is the rationale? And so it was that I reminded myself again to reflect. And I continue to reflect upon the culture of my own training and how we form habits that seem so straightforward, and they were perhaps in that setting. But more than occasionally, we just might need to be reminded to turn around to face the patient, the woman, as she is, where she is, and see respect with a new lens.

Index